dementia care nursing

promoting well-being in people with dementia and their families

edited by

trevor adams

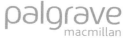

palgrave
macmillan

First published in 2008 by
PALGRAVE MACMILLAN
Houndmills, Basingstoke, Hampshire RG21 6XS and
175 Fifth Avenue, New York, N.Y. 10010
Companies and representatives throughout the world.

PALGRAVE MACMILLAN is the global academic imprint of the Palgrave
Macmillan division of St. Martin's Press, LLC and of Palgrave Macmillan Ltd.
Macmillan® is a registered trademark in the United States, United Kingdom
and other countries. Palgrave is a registered trademark in the European
Union and other countries.

ISBN-13: 978–1–4039–1651–8
ISBN-10: 1–4039–1651–9

This book is printed on paper suitable for recycling and made from fully
managed and sustained forest sources. Logging, pulping and manufacturing
processes are expected to conform to the environmental regulations of
the country of origin.

A catalogue record for this book is available from the British Library.

10 9 8 7 6 5 4 3 2 1
17 16 15 14 13 12 11 10 09 08

Printed and bound in China

This book is dedicated to my two sons Thomas and Jonathan

Contents

List of tables and figures

Tables

Figures

Living longer – if not living forever – is part of the neurosis of our time. Indeed, having a *long* life as opposed to living life fully, productively, creatively and meaningfully has become something of an obsession, except perhaps for those who are poor, ill, disadvantaged or oppressed. Dr Johnson said of the man who knows he is to be hanged in a fortnight, 'it concentrates his mind wonderfully'. Clearly many people are too busy staying alive or staying solvent to worry about living for an eternity.

At the same time a strange infatuation with youth and youthfulness is abroad in the land. Many of my baby-boomer contemporaries give surgeons free rein to nip and tuck them, or let style gurus rampage through their wardrobes, all in a vain effort to stay young. Indeed it is doubly vain. Nothing lasts in our ephemeral universe and, like Narcissus, our self-love may eventually be our downfall.

These yearnings may not be central to this book's agenda but undoubtedly are part of the reason for it being written. The longer we live, the more people will develop one form of dementia or another. We live in hope of a 'cure' being just around the corner, but that too might be part of the adolescent fantasies that rule our lives. We find it difficult to confront our mortality. We shy away from acknowledging that we will not live forever, or if we do live to a ripe age, it might be with sorely depleted physical or mental resources. That scares us. Better not to dwell on it. And so we focus on the ephemeral 'here and now' and play at being youthful.

To what extent are these fantasies about longevity and youth part of the problem of dementia care? I suspect that my question will be answered indirectly in this book. Our society's problem with ageism reflects the widespread fear of death. Our fashionable embrace of youth 'culture', in its myriad forms, is merely part of our denial of ageing and decay. That said, it is worth remembering that not all societies are afflicted with ageism. Globalisation, and its attendant materialist values, may pose a threat but many cultures still value age as a possible source of wisdom. Where we might view our political leaders as 'too old' at 60, other societies might worry that 70 is still 'too young'. Whether we shall ever reverse the current devaluation of the aged person is another 'big question'. However, by talking about age, life experience and the practical business of 'gaining wisdom', we might begin to question the absolute value of youth and youthfulness.

Although written for professionals involved in the delivery of dementia care the book's content is relevant to everyone, at some point in their lives. However, perhaps only a direct encounter with dementia will make us want to *study* this book carefully, so that we might learn something of meaningful value. Until we have such an encounter – whether as a professional, family member or friend – we can hold dementia at bay, maintaining it as an academic topic, not really meaningful in the context of our lives.

When my mother developed dementia a decade ago my family were thrown into a whirlpool of emotional confusion. Our struggle to understand what was happening to her was confused further by the apparent meaningfulness of what professionals saw only as 'bizarre' or 'pathological' behaviour. At the same time we struggled with feelings of guilt, regret, anger and frustration, as we tried to support her on what appeared to be the last stage of her life. In truth this was also another vital stage in our life – as a family. Life was writing important new pages in the storybooks of our own, individual lives. What did we learn about 'dementia' over those five long years? Probably not a lot, since we already had a good 'academic' understanding of the concept. However, as a family, we learned much about our mother, and a little of her experience of the slow dimming of her light. Hopefully, we learned a lot more about ourselves, as persons. If dementia took hold of my mother, it also held up a mirror in which all her family and friends had a chance to see themselves, for the weak, helpless yet remarkably fortunate people we are.

We also learned a lot about caring from that five-year encounter, not least because it often seemed to be in such short supply. Caring – the exercise of compassion, flavoured with altruism – is often seen as uniquely human. Now we know that many of our primate cousins make bountiful displays of altruism and compassion, which differ little from our own. Although it is easy to see our human reflection in the gaze of the apes, other animals are probably no less inclined to generously support their own kin. We simply have not got around to recognising this, 'scientifically'. What does seem self-evident is that humans are losing their capacity to 'care', in any forthright, fundamentally compassionate and 'ordinary' manner. A Scottish university will, later this year, mount a novel programme in 'caring' for nurses, sponsored by a former nurse who made a fortune in the world of transport. To the absolute outsider this must seem like offering artists a course in how to hold a pencil. However, if our experience of the 'care' our mother received is not to be dismissed as extraordinary, perhaps people with ambitions to become nurses need to be taught how to hold that caring pencil.

All of which makes the title of this book – 'Dementia *Care* Nursing' – all the more inspiring. No pussyfooting around with complex neologisms. Let us remind ourselves that the 'extraordinarily ordinary' business of supporting people in their moment of need is called 'caring'. Such an acknowledgement might be another brick in rebuilding the caring base of nursing for the twenty-first century.

I hope that all readers will see much of themselves in the dementia care nursing described in these pages. Having read it, I hope that they will feel better equipped to navigate the difficult waters of bureaucracy and prejudice that swirls around the field. But most of all, I hope that they will gain a deeper insight into their own fears, prejudices and deep-brooding ignorance about the people – and their loved ones – who are caught in the blinding headlights of dementia.

PROFESSOR PHIL BARKER
Trinity College Dublin and
University of Dundee

This book is concerned with nursing people with dementia and their family members. This is an important issue whose significance must surely increase as many of us live into old age. The book sees dementia care nursing as primarily a practical activity, as something that nurses say and do with people who have dementia and their informal carers. However, the book also argues that nursing practice is itself underpinned by ideas, theories and evidence that guide and direct exactly what it is that nurses say and do. Thus, the book develops an integrated and balanced approach that recognises the mutual and reciprocal contribution of theory and practice in dementia care nursing.

I first became aware of dementia in 1972, when I visited the wife of a clergyman I was staying with. I found the visit very distressing. The ward was bleak, institutional and smelt! However, I was amazed by the love and care the man showed his wife. A few years later in 1978, I was training to be a mental health nurse and was allocated to a geriatric ward. The ward was slightly more welcoming than the ward I had experienced a few years earlier but it was still pretty awful. However, it was on that ward that I became interested in nursing people with dementia. When I qualified as a nurse I was asked which ward I wanted to work on. The Senior Nurse was amazed when I said that I wanted to work with older people and thought there must be something wrong with me! In today's language, it simply was not cool to work with older people.

There have been many changes in the way people, some people at least, think about people with dementia. We have to thank Tom Kitwood for helping nurses and other health and social workers see people with dementia as actually what they are – people. His death, at a relatively early age was a great loss. While his ideas have had a great influence on dementia care, it would be inappropriate not to move on and develop his work further and build on it to help nurses understand more fully the experience of people with dementia and their informal carers.

It is very easy to imagine that just because Kitwood's ideas have dominated dementia care for the past ten years that all dementia care units and all nursing homes employ his ideas (Kitwood, 1997). I wish that this was the case! As the Rowan Report (CHI, 2003) indicated, there are many places in the United Kingdom that are just as institutional as the wards I saw more than thirty years ago. It would be very easy to hide poor care within a smoke screen of person-centred care and think person-centred care happens on every ward. It does not.

This book draws on more recent work in Nursing that challenges some of the ideas that Kitwood put forward. The book draws on relationship-centred approaches to care that recognise that other people are involved in the provision of dementia care and that the relationship between each party affects the quality of care (Nolan et al., 2004; Adams, 2005; Adams and Gardiner, 2005). The book also draws upon various writers who recognise the importance of the body within dementia care and acknowledges how people's experience of dementia is both a bodily and embodied experience (Phinney and Chesla, 2003; Kontos, 2006). This is something that Kitwood's work did not really do. Finally, the book draws on the work of activity theory together with the work of the philosopher Margaret Archer (2000) that highlights the contribution made by bodily activity and shows how it gives rise to people's sense of selfhood. This is a somewhat different approach to Kitwood, who argues that the personhood of people with dementia arises out of other people's interaction with them. The book takes an integrated and balanced approach and argues that identity arises from what people say and do to those with dementia. Thus, the book does not dismiss Kitwood's work but rather integrates his views with more recent insights and so allows nurses to have a much broader view of dementia care.

The book's development did not just lie in academic argument and reflection. Various issues have happened in my own life that have contributed to its development. Not least among these was the onset of my mother's dementia. I had just come to see how having someone in the family with dementia affects all the family, when my mother developed dementia herself. I did not realise that she had dementia at first but thought it was her diabetes. My mother's dementia happened very quickly and within a few months of its onset, she had severe dementia and was in a nursing home. I found it very difficult to look at my mother's face and think that it was her. It made me feel so sad to think of who she once was and who she had become. I had not had a very good relationship with my stepfather; it was neither his fault nor mine. Through this time I came to more fully understand that 'dementia was a family affair'. I learnt to develop a much better relationship with my step-father, and so after my mother died, five years later, my step-father came to my wedding and later gave gifts to my children on behalf of my mother. Relationships certainly do matter.

It has recently come to light that the amount of attention nurses on pre-registration nursing programmes give towards learning skills that are specifically directed towards enhancing the physical, psychological and social well-being of people with dementia and their families is appallingly low (Chang et al., 2005; Pulsford et al., 2007). Nursing Education is just as ageist as the rest of the nursing profession and this is just not acceptable. It is hoped that the book will help contribute towards a new understanding of dementia care nursing and lead to it being seen as an interesting and worthwhile area of nursing practice. However, the book will be particularly helpful for nurses taking undergraduate and postgraduate qualifications in which there is a component on dementia care. While the book is primarily intended for nurses, its development of theory in dementia care, from a person-centred and relationship-centred approach to a whole systems approach provides a critical approach that may make the book worthwhile reading for other professional groups working with people who have dementia and their families.

Many people have contributed towards this book, though most of them probably do not realise it! I would like to thank the anonymous reviewers for their helpful comments about the first draft of this book. I want to thank Professor Karen Bryan, Head of Division, Division of Health and Social Care, Faculty of Health & Medical Sciences, University of Surrey, who is a specialist in communication and dementia care and who is always ready to discuss ideas and read papers that I have written. Some parts of this book were written while I was on a study visit to Australia. I also want to thank Professor Wendy Moyle, Deputy Director of the Research Centre for Clinical Practice Innovations, Griffith University, Brisbane, Queensland, for giving me the opportunity to spend time at Griffith University. I also want to thank Professor Helen Bartlett, Director, Australasian Centre on Ageing, University of Queensland and Professor Rhonda Nay, La Trobe University, Melbourne, for allowing me to spend time in their Departments and share ideas about dementia care nursing. I also want to thank Professor Jenny Abbey, Professor of Nursing (Aged Care), Queensland University of Technology, for the help and interest she has shown in my work. Thanks also go to Coombe Healthcare, Rosemary Park, Haslemere, for supporting the Oldercare Practice Development Project that allowed me to spend a considerable amount of time observing how nurses work with people who have dementia. I would like to thank the editorial staff at Palgrave Macmillan, Lynda Thompson and Sarah Lodge, for their help and support. I would like to thank my wife, Helena for the care and attention she has given to indexing the book. I would also like to thank the many students I have taught at the University of Surrey, particularly those undertaking specialist modules in dementia care on undergraduate and postgraduate programmes. I am also indebted to those people with dementia that I have nursed and their families for sharing their lives with me and helping me understand what it means to nurse people with dementia.

TREVOR ADAMS
University of Surrey
Guildford UK
July 2007

References

Adams, T. (2005). From person-centred care to relationship-centred care. *Generations Review* 15, 1, 4–7.

Adams, T. and Gardiner, P. (2005). Communication and interaction within dementia care triads: developing a theory for relationship-centred care. *Dementia* 4, 2, 185–205.

Archer, M. (2000). *Being Human: The Problem of Agency.* Cambridge: Cambridge University Press.

Chang, E., Hancock, K., Harrison, K., Daly, J., Johnson, A., Easterbrook, S., Noel, M., Luhr-Taylor, M. and Davidson, P. M. (2005). Palliative care for end-stage dementia: A discussion of the implications for education of health care professionals. *Nurse Education Today* 25, 4, 326–332.

CHI (2003). *Investigations Arising from Care on Rowan Ward Manchester Mental and Social Care Trust*. London: TSO.

Kitwood, T. (1997). *Dementia Reconsidered*. Buckingham: Open University Press.

Kontos, P. C. (2006). Embodied selfhood: the expression of ethnographic of Alzheimer's disease. In A. Leibing and L. Cohen (eds) *Thinking about Dementia: Culture, Loss and the Anthropology of Senility*. New Brunswick: Rutgers University Press, pp. 195–217.

Nolan, M. R., Davies, S., Brown, J., Keady, J. and Nolan, J. (2004). Beyond 'person-centred' care: a new vision for gerontological nursing. *Journal of Clinical Nursing* 13, s1, 45–53.

Phinney, A. and Chesla, C. A. (2003). The lived body in dementia. *Journal of Aging Studies* 17, 285–299.

Pulsford, D., Hope, K. and Thompson, R. (2007). Higher education provision for professionals working with people with dementia: A scoping exercise. *Nurse Education Today* 27, 1, pp. 5–13.

Trevor Adams, MSc PhD RGN RMN Cert Ed. CPN Cert.
Dr Trevor Adams is Lecturer in Mental Health, University of Surrey. His PhD studied the relationship between people with dementia, family carers and dementia care nurses. He has nursed people with dementia and their families in hospitals and the community. Trevor has spoken widely at conferences in the United Kingdom and abroad and has co-authored *Dementia Care: Developing Partnerships in Practice* with Charlotte Clarke (Baillière Tindal), *Dementia Care* with Jill Manthorpe (Arnold) and *Community Mental Health Nursing and Dementia Care: Practice Perspectives* with John Keady and Charlotte Clarke (Open University Press). Trevor was Committee Member of Royal College of Nursing Mental Health and Older People Forum (2004–2006) and was External Examiner, BSc (Hons) Dementia Studies, University of Bradford (2003–2006).

Elizabeth Anderson, BA (Hons) MSc DPhil
Dr Elizabeth Anderson leads modules at both the undergraduate and postgraduate level on courses in Dementia Studies run by the Bradford Dementia Group. She completed her DPhil. thesis at the University of Oxford in 1999, and building on this work, has published in the area of understanding and assessing memory change in older people. More recently, she has become interested in the implications of brain–behaviour relationships for understanding people with dementia and their care needs, rather than simply understanding dementia.

Tula Brannelly, BPhil PhD RMN PG Cert Ed.
Dr Tula Brannelly is Senior Lecturer in Mental Health Nursing at Massey University, Wellington, New Zealand. Tula has a practice background caring for people with dementia, and her PhD examined the ethical decision-making of Community Psychiatric Nurses and Social Workers using an ethic of care. She has an interest in

researching user perspectives and participation in mental health services, and teaches mental health in undergraduate and postgraduate nursing.

Ingrid Eyers, PhD FHEA MSc RGN
Dr Ingrid Eyers is Lecturer in Adult Nursing, University of Surrey. Her PhD studied the experience and use of emotions in the care of vulnerable older people. At present Ingrid is part of the New Dynamics of Ageing funded SomnIA (Sleep in Ageing) research project where she leads the team researching the determinants of poor sleep amongst older people living in care homes. Ingrid is a member of the British Society of Gerontology Executive Committee and was Honorary Secretary (2005–2007).

Liz Forbat, BA PhD PG Cert.
Dr Liz Forbat is Senior Research fellow at the University of Stirling, leading a programme of research on children and families. Her PhD was a study of caregiving relationships, using discourse analysis to identify the patterns of talk which shed light on troubled relationships. She has published widely and is the author of *Talking About Care: Two sides to the story* (Policy Press) and co-author of *Relating experience: Stories from health and social care* with Caroline Malone, Martin Robb and Janet Seden (Routledge).

Sue Hodge PG Dip (Social Welfare Law) (Leicester)
Sue Hodge was admitted as a solicitor in 1969 but left practice to teach more than 20 years ago. She has taught at law to undergraduate and post-graduate students. She has been associated with the University of Surrey for the past three years and is keen to make the law comprehensible to health care professionals. She is the author of *Tort Law* (Willan Publishing) which is now in its fourth Edition and has co-written *Unlocking Torts* (with Chris Turner, Hodder Press), which is now in its second Edition.

Chapter 1

Nursing with people who have dementia: an introduction

Trevor Adams

Learning Outcomes

After reading this chapter you will be able to

- discuss the possible impact of demographic and epidemiological trends on the incidence of dementia;
- describe clinical features associated with various types of dementia;
- describe what is meant by Critical Realism and its contribution to dementia care nursing;
- describe what is meant by the dialectical approach towards the dementia process;
- outline the contribution of the systemic approach to dementia care nursing.

Introduction

Over the past 30 years, public recognition of dementia has considerably increased. One reason why this has occurred is that there is now an increasing number of people in the world, including the United Kingdom (UK) who have dementia. In 2007, *Dementia UK* (AS, 2007) estimated that there were 683,597 people in the UK with dementia. By 2021, the report argues that this number will increase to 940,110 and is expected to rise to over 1,735,087 million people by 2051. This predicted increase is due to the rise in the number of older people in the UK, particularly those over 85 years, and also the increased risk that older people have of developing dementia. While it is tempting to think in apocalyptic terms of a 'rising tide' of older

people with dementia that is threatening to engulf us, it is more realistic to think that the increase will be more gradual.

There is a second reason why public recognition of dementia has
increased over the past few years. Recent developments within health
and social care have been characterised by a transition from institution-
based to community-based services. Rather than living behind the
walls of an asylum, present social policy asserts that people with
dementia should live in the community and be supported by their
families who in turn receive (hopefully!) support from a wide range
of community-based agencies such as social workers and community
mental health nurses. Thus people with dementia have become more
visible in the community, and frequently remain within the family
and are part of many people's experience of family life.

Dementia is an acquired syndrome that is chronic, progressive
and debilitating. The syndrome is characterised by global impairments that affect higher brain function. People with the syndrome
find it difficult to remember what has happened to them, communicate with other people and undertake skilled social behaviour. While
dementia is usually seen as a memory disorder, it is more accurate to
think of it as comprising a wide range of physical, emotional, behavioural and social phenomena that progressively impair people's
ability to undertake socially accepted activities of everyday life.

The clinical features of dementia comprise memory difficulties,
particularly of recent events; orientation, regarding time, place and
person; grasping items of new information; communication with
other people; personality changes and behaviour disorders. There
are two types of dementia: primary dementia and secondary
dementia. Primary dementias are those that mainly affect the
neurones in the brain, such as in Alzheimer's disease, dementia
with Lewy Bodies (DLB) and other forms of fronto-temporal lobar
atrophies such as Pick's Disease. Secondary dementias are dementias in which damage to neurones is secondary to pathologies in
other tissues. They include vascular or multi-infarct dementia and
dementias that arise from infections, metabolic disorders, nutrition,
traumas and brain tumours.

People with dementia often experience non-cognitive behavioural disorders such as delusions, visual hallucinations, sleep
disturbance, overactivity, aggression and depression. People in the
later stages of Alzheimer's disease may develop hyperrelexia and
apractic gait. Sudden jerking of the head limbs and trunk called
myoclonus occurs in 15% of patients. Alzheimer's disease lasts

between 8 and 10 years, but it can last as little as 2 years and as long as 22 years!

The most common types of dementia are

- Alzheimer's disease
- vascular dementia
- DLB
- fronto-temporal dementia and Pick's disease

Alzheimer's Disease

There are two forms of Alzheimer's disease: an early-onset familial Alzheimer's disease (EOFAD) or a sporadic late onset Alzheimer's disease (LOAD). Each form is characterised by amyloid-containing extracellular plaques and the abnormal material that develop inside the neurone, the neurofibrillary tangles. It has been found that the degeneration of neurones may arise as a result of the deposition of amyloid beta-peptide in the brain. The EOFAD appears linked with three genes on chromosomes 21,14q and 1q. People with Alzheimer's disease have lower levels of acetylcholine in their transmitter fluids between neurones. The clinical features of Alzheimer's disease are typical to those found in the dementia syndrome, though usually it has a slow onset.

Alzheimer's disease is characterised by

- dementia: cognitive decline;
- gradual progression;
- intact level of consciousness;
- onset after the age of 40 years.

A definite diagnosis of 'Alzheimer's disease' is usually only possible after death and comprises impairment to memory (amnesia), co-ordination dexterity (apraxia), language (aphasia) and perception (agnosia). In the early stages of Alzheimer's disease, people experience memory difficulties and may develop personality changes. Later, people with Alzheimer's disease may find difficulty in using language, undertaking everyday activities and recognising people, places and situations. During this stage, family members often help the person by doing such tasks as going for shopping and paying their bills. In the latter stages of Alzheimer's disease people experience severe difficulty with their memory and in recognising other people. They may also have difficulty in walking and toileting, and gradually may become fully dependent on other people for all their activities of daily living.

Vascular Dementia

Vascular dementia is caused by a deficiency of the supply of oxygen to the brain following a stroke or a small vessel disease. The symptoms experienced by the person will depend on the part of the brain that has been damaged. Occasionally vascular dementia may arise as a result of a single stroke and is called 'a single-infarct dementia'. However, it is more common for vascular dementia to arise from a series of small strokes, when it is called 'multi-infarct dementia'. Vascular dementia usually starts abruptly, recurrent small strokes may give rise to a typical step-wise progression, and afterwards multiple infarcts may occur. Focal deficits may also occur and lead to neurological problems. It is easy to distinguish between Alzheimer's disease and vascular dementia. While they are two different conditions, they often occur together, and when this happens they are described as 'a mixed dementia'. Over the past ten years, people have become more aware of different 'new dementias', which until recently have been thought rare. These conditions include Dementia with Lewy Bodies (DLB), fronto-temporal dementia and Pick's disease.

Dementia with Lewy Bodies

Dementia with Lewy bodies may account for between 10% and 15% of all cases of dementia. Lewy bodies are small spherical protein deposits in the nerve cells that disrupt normal functioning of the brain and interrupt the action of neurotransmitters such as acetylcholine and dopamine. Lewy bodies are also found in the brains of people with Parkinson's disease, which is a progressive neurological condition that affects people's movement.

DLB is a progressive condition that typically develops over several years and will have some of the symptoms of Alzheimer's and Parkinson's disease. People with DLB experience memory loss, spatial disorientation and communication difficulties associated with Alzheimer's disease, and slow movements, muscle stiffness, trembling limbs, shuffling gait and mask-like expression associated with Parkinson's disease. There are also a number of symptoms that are specific to DLB, which may include

- abilities fluctuating during the day;
- feeling faint or having 'funny turns';
- experiencing vivid and detailed visual hallucinations;
- sleeping during the day and have restless sleep at night.

Fronto-temporal Dementia and Pick's Disease

The term 'fronto-temporal dementia' covers a range of conditions, including Pick's disease, frontal lobe degeneration and dementia associated with motor neurone disease. All these conditions are caused by damage to the frontal lobe and/or the temporal parts of the brain which are responsible for people's behaviour, emotional responses and language skills.

Fronto-temporal dementia is a rare form of dementia. Younger people, specifically those under the age of 65, are more likely to be affected. Damage to the frontal and temporal lobe areas of the brain causes a variety of different symptoms.

During the initial stages of fronto-temporal dementia, the person is usually less forgetful than in Alzheimer's disease. However, their personality and behaviour may change. These changes may include lack of insight; they may appear selfish and unfeeling and may lose inhibitions – for example, exhibiting sexual behaviour in public. The rate of progression of fronto-temporal dementia varies enormously, ranging from less than two years to over ten years. In the later stages, the damage to the brain is usually more generalised, and symptoms usually appear to be similar to those of Alzheimer's disease. People affected may no longer recognise their friends and family, and may need nursing care.

My Story

Like many people, someone in my family had dementia. In my case, it was my mother. By that time, I had been working with people who had dementia for about ten years and had written two articles on the subject. I remember talking to my mother about the first of these articles which was called *Dementia is a Family Affair* (Adams, 1987). She was pleased that I had written the article, though little did I know that only a year later she would have dementia herself.

I had just moved to London, while my mother, by then, was living about 350 miles away in the North East of England. We had previously lived in Manchester and neither of us had much experience of the North East. She had recently moved there with my stepfather whom she had married when I was 15 years old, about four years after my father had died. Both my mother and I had no brothers and sisters, and so there were no other relatives around.

At the time, I was working in London as a researcher on a project for older people with mental health problems. Every so often, a phone call would come to the Team Leader's office, and she would shout out of her office saying 'Trevor, there's a call for you.' I would then rush over to her office, put the phone to my ear, and hear pip, pip, pip, pip. No answer. This kept happening day after day, and I realised that it was my mother who was trying to ring me. What could I do? She had no phone at home, and I could not phone her back or get in touch with her in the evening. I wanted to know what was wrong with her.

One weekend I was anxious about my mother and I decided to drive up the M1 and see her. It was a long journey and the motorway was covered with snow. News reports had advised people not to make journeys that were not really necessary. There were only a few cars on the road, and everything was cold, white and silent. I eventually made it up the motorway and got to see my mother. We spent a long time talking about what had been happening. She told me about visits to the doctor and different things that had happened. What she told me seemed unreal, slightly exaggerated and strange. I tried to work out what was happening to her, as nurses do, and thought that her confusion was due to her diabetes. She looked thinner and rather dishevelled, and I hoped her doctor was treating it as best he could.

I made the long journey up to the North East quite a few times. Not all of these journeys were in the snow, and on one journey I witnessed a freak display of the Northern Lights. However, every time I went to see my mother, I was filled with a deep discomfort and overwhelming despair about what was happening.

Some sort of breakthrough came when I took my mother to Durham one Sunday. I took her to the Cathedral, a nice and historic place, much nicer than the town where she lived. We were walking along at the back of the Cathedral and she tripped on the stone floor. She got up and I asked her if she was alright. She said she was fine. I then went into the men's toilets and she went to the ladies'. When I came out of the toilet, I waited for my mother to come out, but there was no sign of her. I waited and worried that the fall had caused a sub-arachnoid haemorrhage, and that she was lying on the toilet floor. I felt helpless standing there and did not feel (probably quite wisely!) able to go into the toilets to look for her. I waited for a woman who was going into the toilet. I told her what had happened, and she said that she would look for my mother. However, the woman came out and said that there was no one in the toilet. I then realised that I had lost my mother!

I did not know Durham, and so I ran across the city looking for a phone box. When I found one, I phoned the police; after a few minutes I was picked up by a police car from outside the phone box. Soon a call came over the police radio saying that they had found a woman wandering about inside the Cathedral and that she was with the people giving out hymn books. When I got there, she was confused and had soil over her clothes. I asked her about the soil and she was not able to tell me where it had come from. The people giving out the hymn books seemed angry with me and blamed me for letting her go off on her own. I realised they did not really understand what had happened and I just accepted what they said to me. At that point, probably for the first time, I understood what had happened. My mother had dementia just like all the other people I had seen on the wards and as a community mental health nurse. I had listened to so many people telling me about how their husbands and wives had become confused and had become lost, and now it was happening to my mother.

Within a few weeks, my mother's confusion had worsened, and she went into an assessment unit at the local psychiatric unit to be assessed and then moved on to a nursing home. I found visiting my mother at the home very difficult. When I first saw my mother on a ward with people who had dementia, I cried. I just thought of the juxtaposition between what she was now and how she must have been when she was a child. I felt so sad.

It would have been easier if I had a friend to go with every time. However, I was single at the time and had to make the long and miserable journey on my own. I dreaded seeing her and put it off week after week. I got guilty for not visiting her every weekend and feared hearing the news that she had died and I had not visited her.

Seeing her there, I did not know what to say, and looking at her was so difficult.

After about four years, I got engaged. I took my fiancée to see my mother and told my mother that I was going to get married. I do not know whether my mother understood what I was saying, though my fiancée says she did.

A few weeks later, about five minutes after going into teach a group of students, a fellow teacher came into the class and said he had a message for me. Outside the classroom, he told me that my stepfather had phoned up to tell me that my mother had died. I was devastated. The class was told that I was not available to continue the lesson, and I was given a few days off work to see to things. I went straightway to see a friend, a librarian in a nearby hospital whom I had spoken to many times about my mother, but she was not there. She was not there, but, thankfully, sitting at one of the tables was a teacher with whom I had worked, who was a specialist in grief therapy, and she talked to me about what had happened. I phoned my fiancée and she said that she would come up to the North East for the funeral and that I could stay with her and her family in Devon. After a few days getting used to what had happened, we went up to the North East to attend my mother's funeral.

As someone who teaches dementia care nursing in a university, it is understandable that I value the contribution that research and theory makes to the knowledge nurses use when working alongside people with dementia and their families. However, many of the ideas in this book do not arise from hours of reading academic papers in university libraries but from the time my mother had dementia. During that time, I shared much of the despair many people experience when they have a close relative with dementia. As much as anything else, I learnt that dementia really was a family affair, and that not only was it a mistake to focus on just the person with dementia, but it was also a mistake to focus on just the carer. Over this time, I came to see a much bigger picture in which the experience of the person with dementia was affected by different agencies in society: by nurses and families, hospitals and care agencies, governments and politicians as well as cultural artefacts such as language and the way it constructs situations and places people in different social positions and offers them different experiences, identities, obligations and responsibilities.

The Book

While the book acknowledges the value of recent approaches such as that of Tom Kitwood and recognises their important and seminal impact upon dementia care, it is now time to move 'beyond person-centred care' (Nolan et al., 2004) and adopt a broader approach that widens the view of nurses and allows them to see each person and agency that contributes to the well-being of the person with dementia. One approach that has moved in this direction is 'relationship-centred care' (Nolan et al., 2003; Adams, 2005). This approach identifies the contribution of three people or agencies in the provision of care: the person with dementia, the family carer(s) and the health and social care professional(s), and argues that the quality of care received is associated with the maintenance of good relationships between each of these (Nolan et al., 2004).

In addition, the book applies a particular philosophical approach – Critical Realism – to dementia care nursing. This approach offers dementia care nursing a holistic basis that does not adhere to the traditional division between the natural and social sciences (Bhaskar, 1989). This approach has recently been developed within mental health nursing (Littlejohn, 1993; McEvoy and Richards, 2003) and overcomes the dichotomy between realist and interpretative approaches towards mental health nursing, such as those of Gournay (2000) and Barker (1999, 2001), respectively. Critical Realism argues that there exists an objectively knowable and independent reality, whilst acknowledging the role of perception and cognition in its generation. Thus knowledge is viewed as a social and historical product that is specific to time and place, and is mediated through models, metaphors, discourses and narratives. Critical Realism, therefore, combines a realist ontological perspective (theory of being) with a relativist epistemology (theory of knowledge) (Williams, 1999, 2003). This way of understanding the process of 'knowing' acknowledges the tangible nature of dementia, for example, pathological and behavioural changes (hence 'Realism'), while fully acknowledging that the only way to know about what happens to people with dementia and their family carers is through the use of models, metaphors, discourses and narratives (hence a 'critical' approach to Realism) – that is through the accounts offered by doctors, nurses, relatives and people with dementia themselves.

In terms of nursing practice, Critical Realism offers dementia care nursing a way of fully taking account of physical *and* psycho-social aspects that affect the person with dementia and their families. This approach corresponds well with Kitwood's dialectical understanding of the dementia process (Kitwood, 1997).

Physical/Pathological Processes and Psycho-social Phenomena

People's experience of dementia arises out of an interrelationship between physical/bio-medical and social/psychological phenomena. This influential, dialectical understanding of the dementia process was initially put forward by Kitwood (1997) and has important implications for how care is provided for people with dementia. There has been a temptation, perhaps due to an overreaction to the past excessive medicalisation and institutionalisation of people with dementia to regard the dialectical nature of dementia as only highlighting the contribution of social and psychological phenomena to the dementia process. After reading (and re-reading) his work, it is clear that this is not Kitwood's original understanding of the dementia process, and recent writers have begun to reassert Kitwood's initial assertion about the mutual and dialectical contribution of physical/biomedical and social/ psychological phenomena within the dementia process (see Downs et al., 2006).

As well as allowing the contribution of physical and biomedical contribution to people's experience of dementia, Kitwood's dialectical approach also allows us to understand how dementia is constructed through social interaction (Sabat, 2001, 2006). Within the approach, people with dementia are seen as being like everybody else and located within a matrix of social practices and interpersonal relationships. Through relationships, people with dementia, particularly through what others say and do, are understood to develop a sense of identity and occupy a position within the social order (Antaki and Widdicombe, 1998). We would support this idea but would add that first, the identity of everyone, not just the person with dementia, emerges through reciprocated interaction rather than as it is in Kitwood's work, from what the carer says and does to the person with dementia (Nolan et al., 2004). And second, identity also arises through what people with dementia say and do themselves, that is, through their participation in everyday social activity and through what they are able to accomplish for themselves.

Biological, Family and Cultural Systems

Since people's experience of living with dementia arises through reciprocal relationships and participative activity, it follows that a wide range of people and agencies contribute towards their experience of dementia and their provision of care. We would, therefore, want to adopt a much broader approach than person-centred care and relationship-centred care within dementia care nursing and align dementia care nursing with various approaches that highlight the systemic nature of nursing, such as Family Nursing (Friedman et al., 2003) and Family Systems Nursing (Wright and Leahey, 2005).

Approaches such as these are now an important part of health and social policy and are known as 'the whole systems approach' (DH, 2005a). While we believe that person-centred care and relationship-centred care have an important contribution to make within dementia care nursing, we see them as providing 'a partial view' rather than the whole picture, and would see systemic approaches as providing a more inclusive approach towards dementia care nursing that allows biological and psycho-social aspects of the person with dementia, their family, the health and social care system, voluntary and government agencies to be taken into account.

Structure of the Book

The ideas that have already been described are developed more fully in the forthcoming chapters. Chapter 2 provides a review of the historical and theoretical background to dementia care nursing and develops the view that people with dementia are found within different areas of health care provision, and that dementia care nursing should be the concern of all nurses. This position is supported by the document *Everybody's Business* (DH, 2005a). The chapter continues by defining nursing people with dementia, and identifying different key ideas that underpin its practice.

Over the past 25 years, many new and innovative approaches towards people with dementia have been developed. Perhaps the most important of these is 'person-centred care' developed by Tom

Kitwood (1937–1997). Chapter 3 outlines Kitwood's person-centred approach to people with dementia. Despite the major impact Kitwood's work has had on dementia care, various shortcomings have been identified and are discussed in the chapter. Nevertheless, the chapter reaffirms various aspects of Kitwood's approach, such as his dialectical understanding that integrates bio-medical and psycho-social aspects of the dementia process, and supports the recent elaboration of his approach (Brooker, 2006; O'Connor, 2007). The chapter continues by examining other approaches towards people with dementia, such as those that highlight hearing the voice of a person with dementia, attachment approaches and the early experience of people with dementia. The chapter concludes by arguing that while each of these approaches offer valuable and distinctive insights, they nonetheless, focus only on the person with dementia and neglect other people and agencies that are involved in the provision of dementia care nursing.

In Chapter 4, Elizabeth Anderson examines the biological and physiological changes that occur in people with dementia. In spite of Kitwood's dialectical understanding of the dementia process, personhood has only tended to be represented as resulting from how people talk to people with dementia. This innovative chapter takes a broader view of personhood that reaffirms Kitwood's dialectical understanding of dementia and describes the contribution of neurological aspects to understanding people with dementia. The chapter is of particular value to nurses working with people who have dementia, as nursing practice is often associated with caring for the body and is underpinned by a bio-psycho-social model of health.

Having examined the psycho-social and neurological experience of people with dementia, Chapter 5 critically examines the experience of informal carers of people with dementia. The chapter initially charts the development 'informal care' within health and social policy within the UK and argues that while informal care was incorporated into health and social policy in the 1980s, it continues to be a dominant feature. Owing to the governmental interest in informal care, a substantial amount of empirical research has occurred and has given rise to the emergence of different theoretical approaches such as 'transactional' approaches that highlight different stressors experienced by informal carers. The chapter continues by discussing alternative approaches towards the informal care of people with dementia, such as those concerned with loss and temporal approaches that identify different stages within the process of informal care. The chapter concludes by suggesting that policy and practice that focuses on informal care tend to neglect the person with dementia and lead to a one-sided view of dementia care nursing. Chapter 6 examines different ways of addressing the problem that person-centred care and approaches that focus on the informal carer only really address the needs of the person with dementia and informal carer, respectively. To do this, the chapter examines recent 'dyadic' and 'triadic' approaches towards dementia care that highlight the relationship between the person with demen-tia *and* their informal, and in the case of triadic approaches, their for-mal carer(s) too. This latter approach is an important feature of various approaches towards 'relationship-centred care' such as those that focus on the 'Senses Framework' (Nolan et al., 2004) and those that highlight how one member of the triad may find oneself excluded and marginalised (Adams and Gardiner, 2005). Recently, however, *Everybody's Business* (DH, 2005a) and the two governmen-tal reviews of Mental Health Nursing (DH, 2006a; Scottish Executive, 2006) have advocated a much broader approach than Kitwood's approach to 'person-centred care and 'relationship-centred care' and have advocated the development of a 'whole systems approach'. This chapter concludes by drawing on existing theory and research that support a whole systems approach towards dementia care nursing.

Underpinning this approach is the idea that different people and agencies within the same or different systems communicate with each other and that through this communication people's experi-ence is constructed together with their identity, responsibilities, obligations and social position within the provision of dementia care. Chapter 7 challenges existing approaches towards communi-cation that have frequently been used within dementia care and adopts an alternative approach that focuses on how language, including body language, contributes to people's experience of dementia and dementia care. The chapter draws on various approaches towards communication such as Conversation Analysis (Hutchby and Wooffitt, 1998) and Discourse Analysis (Potter, 1996) that reveal how language constructs different meanings within social settings and offers people identity and social positions that lead to their inclusion and well-being.

Chapter 8 is concerned with assessment in dementia care nursing and offers guidance about how nurses should assess people with dementia and their families. The chapter adopts a 'strengths approach' in which the strengths of the person with dementia are identified as a means of designing a care plan whose aim is to enhance these strengths. One aspect of assessment is to assess whether situations pose a risk. The chapter, therefore, continues by examining the nature of risk in dementia care settings and its assessment. The chapter argues that while real and tangible risks may exist in a particular social setting, the extent to which they are recognised as a risk is socially constructed, and arises out of the stories, narratives and accounts shared between different people associated with the provision of care. The chapter concludes by offering guidance about how nurses should report and communicate details about people with dementia and their informal carers to the other members of the multi-disciplinary team.

Chapter 9 is concerned with highlighting different activities and interventions that nurses may employ alongside people with dementia and their family members. The chapter supports an activity approach towards people with dementia and describes a range of activities nurses may use to promote the well-being of the person with dementia and their informal carers. The chapter describes good practice in developing therapeutic engagement in dementia care nursing and gives particular attention to situations that nurses come across in dementia care nursing, such as supporting people under crisis, diagnosis-sharing, offering support, problem-solving and networking.

While it is readily acknowledged that family members may experience stress and burnout as they provide physical and emotional care to relatives with dementia, it is not so readily acknowledged that nurses may similarly experience stress. In Chapter 10, Ingrid Eyers and Trevor Adams examine the idea of 'emotional labour' developed by Hochschild (1983) and examine how it may be applied to dementia care nursing. The chapter continues by advocating that all dementia care nurses should have regular clinical supervision and describe how it may be used to help them resolve negative feelings and perceptions about particular aspects of their work.

Chapter 11 describes various clinical settings in which nurses may find themselves working with people who have dementia and their family members. The chapter examines various capabilities, competences and skills that nurses should have to work with people who have dementia. The chapter argues that capabilities and competencies should not be seen as standing alone and should always arise out of a particular theoretical approach. The chapter continues by integrating competencies that have been advocated should be possessed by all registered mental health nurses, in *Best Practice Competencies and Capabilities for Pre-registration Mental Health Nurses in England* (DH, 2006a) with the whole systems approach developed in this book.

Throughout the book, the link between policy and practice is highlighted, and whilst the book has focussed on developing a whole systems approach we would argue that person-centred care and relationship-centred care fit within this broader approach. In Chapter 12, Liz Forbat looks at the idea of relationship-centred care and its relationship to dementia care nursing, and argues that while practice and policy seem to focus on person-centred approaches, academia has focused on how relationships develop within dementia care. She argues that social policy needs to now move beyond an individualised understanding of what it means to be involved in a care relationship and grapple with the complexities of multi-layered relationships.

While whole systems approaches towards dementia care nursing bring into vision different people and agencies that are involved in the provision of nursing, they do raise problems. One particular problem is concerned with whose views, accounts and stories should nurses accept within practice situations: the views of the person with dementia, the views of different family members and friends or the views of different health and social care workers. This important issue is discussed in Chapter 13 by Tula Brannelly as she draws upon post-modern approaches towards nursing ethics as a basis for relationship-centred dementia care nursing. In the chapter she applies theories from caring and political philosophies to dementia care nursing, and through the use of imagined narrative practitioners' voices have been brought together to emphasise the way decisions about ethically difficult and complex situations are made that promote empowerment rather than oppressive forms of care for people with dementia and their carers.

One of the ideas that underpin the whole systems approach is that unlike person-centred care and relationship-centred care, the experience of the person with dementia, their social position and their ability to make decisions is affected by what is happening in other systems. In Chapter 14, Sue Hodge looks at one such system that has immense importance for people with dementia – the legal system. The chapter gives particular attention to the Mental Capacity Act 2005 in the England and Wales, and the implications it has for dementia care nursing, including how the Act understands mental capacity and how it may be tested. This is a very important issue for dementia care nursing as it sets it within a legal framework and gives guidance about the extent to which people with dementia have the right to make their own decisions within nursing settings and clarifies the responsibility nurses have to provide acceptable care.

The last chapter, Chapter 15, provides an overview of the ideas and arguments that are developed throughout the book and discusses their implications for the development of dementia care nursing.

References

Adams, T. (1987). Dementia is a family affair. *Community Outlook*, Feb., 7–8.

Adams, T. (2005). From person-centred care to relationship-centred care. *Generations Review* 15, 1, 4–7.

Adams, T. and Gardiner, P. (2005) Communication and Interaction within dementia care triads: developing a theory for relationship-centred care. *Dementia* 4, 2, 185–205.

Alzheimer's Society. (2007). *Dementia in the UK: the Full Report.* Alzheimer's Society: London.

Antaki, C. and Widdicombe, S. (1998). Identity as an achievement and as a tool. In C. Antaki and S. Widdicombe (eds) *Identities in Talk.* London: Sage, pp. 1–14.

Barker, P. (1999). *The Philosophy and Practice of Psychiatric Nursing.* Edinburgh: Churchill Livingstone.

Barker, P. (2001). The tidal model: the lived-experience in person-centred mental health nursing care. *Nursing Philosophy* 2, 213–223.

Bhaskar, R. (1989). *Reclaiming Reality: a Critical Introduction to Contemporary Philosophy.* London: Verso.

Brooker, D. (2006). *Person Centred Care.* London: Jessica Kingsley.

Department of Health (2005a). *Everybody's Business: Integrated Mental Health Services for Older Adults. A Service Development Guide.* London: Care Services Improvement Partnership (CSIP).

Department of Health (2006a). *From Values to Action: The Chief Nursing Officer's Review of Mental Health Nursing*. London: Department of Health.

Downs, M., Clare, L. and Mackenzie, J. (2006). Understandings of dementia: explanatory models and their implications for the person with dementia and their therapeutic effect. In J. C. Hughes., S. J. Louw and S. R. Sabat (eds) *Dementia: Mind, Meaning and the Person*. Oxford: Oxford University Press, pp. 235–258

Friedman, M. M., Vicky, R., Bowden, V. R. and Jones, E. (2003) Family Nursing: Research, Theory and Practice 5th Edition. Englewood Cliffs: Prentice Hall.

Gournay, K. (2000). Role of the community psychiatric nurse in the management of schizophrenia. *Advances in Psychiatric Treatment* 6, 243–251.

Hochschild, A. R. (1983). *The Managed Heart: Commercialisation of Human Feeling*. Berkeley, CA: University of California Press.

Hutchby, I. and Wooffitt, R. (1998) *Conversation Analysis: Principles, Practice and Applications*. Polity: Cambridge.

Littlejohn, C. (2003). Critical realism and psychiatric nursing: a philosophical inquiry. *Journal of Advanced Nursing* 43, 5, 449–456

McEvoy, P. and Richards, D. (2003). Critical realism: a way forward for evaluation research in nursing? *Journal of Advanced Nursing* 43, 4, 411–420.

Nolan, M. R., Davies, S., Brown, J., Keady, J. and Nolan, J. (2004). Beyond 'person-centred' care: a new vision for gerontological nursing. *Journal of Clinical Nursing* 13, s1, 45–53.

O'Connor, D., Phinney, A., Smith, A., Small, J., Purves, B., Perry, J., Drance, E., Donnelly, M., Chaudhury, H. and Beattie, L. (2007). Personhood in dementia care: developing a research agenda for broadening the vision. *Dementia: The International Journal of Social Research and Practice* 6, 1, 121–142.

Potter, J. (1996). *Representing Reality: Discourse, Rhetoric and Social Construction*. London: Sage.

Scottish Executive. (2006). *Rights, Relationships and Recovery*. Edinburgh: Scottish Executive.

Sabat, S. (2001). *The Experience of Alzheimer's Disease – Life through a Tangled Veil*. Oxford: Blackwell.

Sabat, S. (2006). Mind, meaning and personhood in dementia. In J. C. Hughes., S. J. Louw and S. R. Sabat (eds) *Dementia: Mind, Meaning and the Person*. Oxford: Oxford University Press, pp. 287–302.

Williams, S. J. (1999). Is anybody there? Critical realism, chronic illness and the disability debate. *Sociology of Health and Illness* 21, 6, 797–819.

Williams, S. J. (2003). Beyond meaning, discourse and the empirical world: critical realist reflections on health. *Social Theory and Health* 1, 42–71.

Wright, L. M. and Leahey, M. (2005). *Nurses and Families: A Guide to Family Assessment and Intervention.* (4th ed.) Philadelphia, PA: F. A. Davis Company.

Chapter 2

Nursing people with dementia and their family members

Trevor Adams

Learning Outcomes

After reading this chapter you will be able to

- explain what is meant by dementia care nursing;
- explore the historical development of dementia care nursing;
- outline the governmental policy towards dementia care nursing;
- describe what constitutes 'good practice' in dementia care nursing;
- discuss key ideas that underpin dementia care nursing.

Introduction

The last chapter described how demographic and epidemiological trends in Western society indicate that there will be a rise in the number of older people with dementia. As a result, there is an urgent need to develop services for older people with dementia and that they contain a sufficient number of appropriately trained and experienced nurses. Underlying this book is the view that it is now necessary to address this issue and to critically examine the nature of dementia care nursing, not least who should give it, who should receive it and what it should be like.

Nursing People with Dementia

The book argues that nursing people with dementia is a practical activity and is best understood as something that nurses say and do. Adopting such a practice-orientated approach displays a distrust of some areas of nurse academia that put forward theories about nursing that are out of step with what practising nurses actually do and answers questions that nurses never ask. However, we would not want nurses to take a totally atheoretical and pragmatic approach, and we would suggest that nurses should think deeply about their practice and reflect about clinical situations in which they work.

Dementia Care Nursing – Is It a Nursing Speciality?

People sometimes think that nursing people with dementia is a speciality, and often that it is part of Mental Health Nursing. There are considerable difficulties with this view, as it tends to make nurses working with people who have dementia on general units feel as though they are outsiders to dementia care and that they do not have the right skills to work with people who have dementia. For nurses not working on a specialist dementia unit, people with dementia are usually seen as 'other people's business'!

We would challenge this view and suggest that dementia care nursing is not just undertaken by one particular branch of Nursing, and would argue that it overlaps Adult, Mental Health and Learning Disability Nursing and may occur in a variety of clinical situations such as hospitals, the community and residential nursing homes. Nurses in each of these repeatedly find themselves working with people who have dementia and their families. This view is supported by *Everybody's Business* (DH, 2005a), which asserts that older people with mental health problems, including people with dementia, are found in different areas of health care and that they should have the same expectation of good care as anyone else, including the right to dignity (DH, 2006a) and optimal participation in decision-making. Nursing people with dementia is 'every nurse's business'!

Who's the User and Who's the Carer

An important issue in dementia care nursing is who is the 'user' and who is the 'carer'. These terms are problematic because while everyone agrees that the person with dementia is 'the user' of services, family members providing care are often also seen as users (Gunstone and Robinson, 2007). Moriarty (1999) points out that describing family carers as 'users' can lead carers to take the place of people with dementia and that their views are not sought. This may lead to some people with dementia not having the opportunity to make their views known and fully participate in decision-making. For this reason, this book uses the term 'user' for the person with dementia and the term 'carer' for informal carers such as family members, friends and neighbours.

A (very) Brief History of Dementia Care Nursing
Dementia Care and Institutionalisation

There are very few accounts of people living with dementia before the introduction of community care in the 1950s and 1960s. The literature that is available suggests that most people with dementia found themselves living outside mainstream society in mental hospitals, asylums and institutions and that they soon became 'forgotten people'. Goffman (1965) in his classic study of mental hospitals shows how inmates were managed and controlled through social practices that manipulated their identity and subordinated them to the control of the hospital. These practices led people with dementia, like other inmates to become silent, hidden and powerless in society and unable to make their views and opinions known.

An important way people with dementia were understood by psychiatrists before the 1950s and 1960s was through 'the cognitive paradigm' (Berrios and Freeman, 1990). Throughout the nineteenth and twentieth centuries, people with dementia were seen as having a condition that primarily affected their cognition and gave rise to progressive and inexorable memory failure. However, this way of viewing people with dementia saw them as having no sense of self or personhood (Kitwood, 1997). Examples of how services depersonalised people with dementia may be seen in written documents from that time. Sheldon's (1948) influential report *The Social Medicine of Old Age* for example, says that older people with dementia exhibit a ' ... neglect of excretory habits, causing great domestic difficulties over the extra washing involved; extreme forgetfulness; confusion and a failure in grasp of their surroundings, leading to them to do foolish things and to fail to recognise people' (pp. 124–125). When people with dementia are represented as foolish and forgetful, particularly by such an important and authoritative document, a particular way of thinking about people with dementia is made available which may encourage some nurses and other professionals to think that it is acceptable to treat people with dementia as having no mind and as if they were not really human. Once this occurs, people with dementia, not least because of their cognitive impairment, will often find it difficult to challenge the negative and dehumanising actions of others and affirm their self-hood. This additional social consequence of dementia is called excess disability.

This cognitive understanding of dementia had important consequences for the organisation of nursing care and led to people with dementia being 'warehoused' (Miller and Gwynne, 1972). This occurred when people with dementia were kept or housed for indefinite periods on long-stay wards and was underpinned by the medical model of illness that pervaded mental health care until quite recently, and in many places still does! Warehousing arose because the dominant medical approach viewed people with dementia as having a disease that had no cure. In the absence of a cure, all that could be done was to keep people with dementia in mental hospitals in the hope that one day a cure might be found. Davies (2003) has described care homes employing this approach as 'controlled communities' and notes that within them '[S]afety and containment are the prime objectives ... often at the expense of personalised care, with an overarching and pervasive routine' (p. 232). Moreover, Davies (2003) argues that controlled communities have a detrimental effect on how members of staff communicate with residents. Staff in controlled communities, for example, orientate their daily work to 'getting through' a daily timetable of practical tasks with residents in the shortest possible time, and have little time for spontaneous communication (Norberg et al., 2001). This approach often leads nurses to be unconcerned with the resident's psychosocial well-being.

Before I trained as a nurse in the 1970s, I accompanied a man who was visiting his wife with severe dementia on a long-stay ward for older people in a large mental hospital. The scene on the ward was shocking as gaunt and emaciated women were kept alive and were sitting around with their skirts hoisted three-quarters of the way up their thighs, surrounded by an all-pervasive stench of old urine. It was a horrifying and deeply repulsive sight. The medical model of dementia had little to offer the woman and a state of therapeutic nihilism prevailed.

Insert 2:1 Taken from *In Service of Old Age: the welfare of psychogeriatric patients* **(Whitehead, 1969)**

'Patients were herded together in old, bleak, neglected buildings with large dark wards, closely placed rows of beds, little furniture and frightening inactivity. Multiple regulations curtail the patient's freedoms and reduce their contact with the outside world. They may be confined to the ward and allowed out only in large supervised groups. Privacy, usually valued by the elderly, is often non-existent. Bathing is supervised and may take place in a communal bathroom. Visiting is restricted to a few hours a week and children are often prohibited. To visit some wards for the elderly is to visit the annex to the mortuary. Rows of old people lie in bed with legs bent and muscles wasted by lack of use, eyes dull and vacant, waiting to die'.

Insert 2:2 Taken from *Sans Everything* **(Robb, 1967)**

'[A]fter six months in certain hospitals, there are ways in which psychiatric nurses are no longer like ordinary people. Their attitude to mental illness changes as it does to old age, to cruelty, to people's needs, and to dying. It is as if they become numbed to these things'.

But it was not only the patients who experienced the adverse effects of institutional 'care': warehousing also had a deep and disturbing effect upon many of the staff. In *Sans Everything* (Robb, 1967), a report on the conditions of older people in institutions in the late 1960s, an Acting Chief Male Nurse clearly identified the effect of institutions on its staff (Insert 2:2).

Behind the closed doors of the asylum and out of the view of the wider community, some nurses lost contact with the values and attitudes they had before they worked with people who had dementia. Many staff continued to treat people with dementia like this for many years, and as a recent BBC Panorama programme showed (12 February 2007) some nurses still do.

Mental Health Nursing and People with Dementia

The marginalisation of people with dementia was commonplace in psychiatric nursing before the 1970s. As Professor Tony Butterworth

(1988: p. 39) notes that 'working with elderly confused and dementing patients was, in my own training lifetime, used as a punishment for nurses who had overstepped the mark or committed an organisational misdemeanour'. Marginalisation was endemic and was even upheld in textbooks for student nurses. For example, Houliston (1961: p. 122) states that people with dementia had 'a state of enfeeblement due to disease or decay of the brain' and that '[U]nlike the mental defective who never was normal, the dement was *normal once*' (my emphasis). These ideas even underpinned questions mental nurses were asked in their final state examination. One question in *The Final Examination Paper Question 1928 for Mental Nurses* asked the student nurses to 'Give an account of the mental symptoms that may be met within a case of senile insanity. Discuss the nursing met within a case of senile insanity. Discuss the nursing requirements of senile patients.'

However, it was not just student nurses who were expected to reproduce these views; they were also found in the views of respected contemporary leaders in nursing such as John Greene (see Insert 2:3).

Considerable changes have occurred in the 40 years since Greene's comments. Many of these changes are due to the enthusiasm and commitment of nurses, often without adequate support and the investment of resources. This was made quite clear in the 1990s Review of Mental Health Nursing *Working in Partnership: a collaborative approach to care* (DH, 1994), which clearly stated that 'Mental health nurses working with elderly people perform

---

Insert 2:3 Taken from *The Psychiatric Nurse in the Community Nursing Service* (Greene, 1968: pp. 177–178)

'The people with dementia can be very uncooperative with members of their own family, but a nurse who has actually known the patient in hospital and seen many similar ones can demonstrate how they can be encouraged for example to take a regular bath and do many things for themselves. Selfishness, greed and so on are not always understood by relatives and a simple explanation of the psychology of old age can be of help. The family is also more likely to cope if they know that the nurse will make regular visits and arrange admission to hospital if the situation gets out of hand. This can provide a period of relief for both the patient and the relatives'.

valuable work, but we found evidence of under investment in training, support and supervision for nursing staff in relation to the very complex and demanding needs of those suffering from dementia' (DH, 1994: p. 34).

Though institutionalisation still remains in some places, the move away from warehousing and institutional forms of dementia care began in the late 1960s. These developments were initiated by a small group of innovative psychiatrists such as Tom Aire and Tony Whitehead who generated professional and academic interest in the provision of services to older people with mental health conditions and gave rise to new models of service delivery, most notably community mental health teams for older people. Whitehead (1970) describes such a team at Severalls Hospital, Essex, comprising different health and social care professionals under the leadership of a Consultant Psychiatrist. Owing to the growing interest in the care of people with dementia within various health and social care professions, different insights and approaches emerged about the physical and emotional well-being of people with dementia and their family members.

Innovation continued throughout the 1980s and 1990s as society became increasingly aware of the rising number of older people with dementia. During this time, mental health nursing services to people with dementia were developed on the basis of the prevailing philosophy of community care and were mainly aimed at supporting the people within their own homes and preventing long-stay hospital admission. These services included the development of day hospitals, respite care and community mental health nursing, many of which were aimed at people with dementia.

This focus on older people did not last for very long and by the late 1990s leading academic mental health nurses were engaged in a programme of refocusing mental health nursing (Repper et al., 1995). The main aim of this project was to raise the focus of working with people who have severe and enduring mental health problems and lowering that of people with short-term disorders who were rather disparagingly called 'the worried well'. While this approach claimed to refocus attention on to people with psychoses, it was only really interested in younger people with functional psychoses such as mania and schizophrenia, not older people with organic psychoses, such as dementia. The approach seemed unaware that dementia is just as much a severe and enduring mental health condition as schizophrenia. As a result of refocusing, services for younger people with severe mental illness (SMI) came to lead the agenda and attract increased funding, and innovative psycho-social interventions (PSI) began to be formulated, tested and form part of the work of many mental health nurses. These services and interventions, however, largely followed an ageist agenda and typically did not deal with older people who had dementia. Refocusing mental health nursing was a setback to mental health nurses working with people who have dementia and from which it still has to recover. Some nurses, however, went beyond the idea of refocusing mental health nursing and supported the development of generic mental health workers and thus lost touch with their historic and distinctive roots within nursing.

At the same time, important and radical changes were emerging in the way people viewed people with dementia and their care. A key idea here was that people with dementia began to be regarded as *people* rather than a mere diagnosis. This holistic approach emphasised that while people with dementia may have lost some cognition, they are still people. These ideas were initially developed by Kitwood (1997), who argued that care staff such as nurses should undertake activities that promote the personhood of people with dementia (see Chapter 3).

Of particular relevance to the recent development of services is *National Service Framework [NSF] for Older People* (DH, 2001). This document is one of a number of frameworks in the United Kingdom (UK) that seek to enhance the provision of care by establishing various national standards. *NSF for Older People* (DH, 2001) comprises eight standards, each relating to different areas of older people's nursing. One of these (and only one!), Standard 7, deals with the mental health of older people. While the needs of people with dementia were addressed in Standard 7, various agencies have argued that older people with dementia received insufficient attention in *The NSF for Older People* (DH, 2001) and led to the marginalisation of people with dementia. However, this marginalisation was compounded by the failure of the *NSF for Mental Health* (DH, 1999) to address the needs of people over the age of 65 years.

The marginalisation of the older people from the *NSF for Mental Health* (DH, 1999) NSFs did not lead to the needs of people with dementia being highlighted and as a result, people with dementia fell through the net and disappeared out of sight. The lack of attention given to older people with dementia in the *NSF for Mental Health*

(DH, 1999) within the context of the expected rise in the number of older people with dementia is a considerable concern together with are a considerable concern. However, the situation is even more alarming as seemingly progress in achieving these Standards is slow. The Healthcare Commission (2006) in its report *Living Well in Later Life* on the first five years of the ten-year plan set out by the *National Service Framework for Older People* (DH, 2001) identifies various areas in which there has been a lack of progress and recommends that further action is still required in three particular areas:

- tackling age discrimination and increased awareness of other diversity areas;
- ensuring that all the standards of the NSF are met including further guidance of implementing the next steps of the NSF from the Department of Health in April 2006;
- strengthening the partnership between all agencies that provide services to older people to ensure that they work together to improve the experiences of older people who use these services.

It is quite clear that a substantial amount of work needs to be undertaken to ensure that the standards set out in the *NSF for Older People* are achieved by 2011.

Failing to highlight the needs of people with dementia was a clear mistake in the NSFs and has contributed towards the continuation of poor standards of care for people with dementia. The poor standards on one ward, Rowan Ward, Withington Hospital, Manchester, attracted the attention of the Commission for Health Improvement (CHI) in October 2003, though it is probably unfair to single out one ward as exhibiting bad practice, as it may well have been happening elsewhere. The Report, *Investigations Arising from Care on Rowan Ward Manchester Mental and Social Care Trust* (CHI, 2003) identified different areas of bad practice that had occurred on Rowan Ward and outlined various circumstances that had brought it about:

- geographical location;
- low staffing levels;
- lack of training;
- lack of nursing leadership;
- lack of clinical governance.

The publication of the Report sent shock waves among health and social care managers and professionals working with people who have dementia, and led the Department of Health to take urgent action to make sure that the same things would never happen again.

One action was to bridge the gap between mental health and dementia care that had been created within government health and social policy. This was accomplished through the joint publication of *Securing Better Mental Health for Older Adults* (DH, 2005b) by the National Directors for Older People and Mental Health. The document provides a vision for how all mainstream health and social care services, with the support of specialist services, should work together to secure better mental health for older adults, and describes how the Department of Health aims to help its implementation.

Everybody's Business

Following the publication of *Securing Better Mental Health for Older Adults* (DH, 2005a), a second more substantial document *Everybody's Business* was published (DH, 2005a). This latter document is a service development guide that lays out the main components of modern services for older people with mental health conditions.

The message put forward by *Everybody's Business* is best summarised in key messages outlined for service commissioners (see Insert 2:4).

Insert 2:4 Summary of key points in *Everybody's Business* (DH 2005)

1. Older people's mental health is everybody's business

Everybody's Business points out that mental health problems in older people are common and that the number of older people in the United Kingdom will rise. In relationship to Alzheimer's disease, which is the commonest form of dementia, th document asserts that the direct cost of Alzheimer's disease exceeds the combined cost of care to society for people who have strokes, cancer and heart disease.

Insert 2:4 cont'd

2. Improving services for older people with mental health problems will help meet national targets and standards

The implication is that forward-looking strategies can improve outcomes for service users and family carers and may generate savings by improving the efficiency of health and social care services. Moreover, *Everybody's Business* commends ways of improving well-being in older people that will support the delivery of a number of national targets and core standards.

3. Access to mental health services should not be based on age

Everybody's Business affirms the idea that people should receive a care that is based on their need, rather than their age. Implicit within this idea is a commitment to services that is user rather than service led and that older people with mental health problems may have needs that require specialist services.

4. Older people need holistic care in mainstream services

This acknowledges that older people with mental health problems may also have physical and mental health needs and the expectation should be that these are addressed appropriately. Moreover, *Everybody's Business* affirms that services should maximise the independence and well-being of older people and their family carers. Finally, there is an understanding that older people with mental disorders should, like anybody else, receive care within mainstream services.

5. Workforce development is central to driving service improvement

Everybody's Business affirms that the problems experienced by people with mental disorders are complex and asserts that there is a need for workforce development, education and training. It also affirms that mainstream staff should be included in training programmes concerned with older people who have mental disorders.

6. Whole system commissioning and leadership are vital to delivering a comprehensive service

Everybody's Business affirms that a co-ordinated approach should be adopted towards older people with mental health problems that integrate health and social care with physical and mental health services and that links should exist also with the housing sector and the voluntary sector.

Everybody's Business has been supplemented by *NICE Clinical Guideline 42* (NICE, 2006) that provides a comprehensive review of multi-disciplinary guidelines for practice within dementia care.

From Values to Action (DH, 2006) and Rights, Relationships and Recovery (Scottish Executive, 2006)

In April 2006, the Chief Nursing Officer at the Department of Health published a review of the work of mental health nurses entitled *From Values to Action* that sought to identify how the profession can best contribute to the care of service users. At the same time, the Chief Nursing Officer of Scotland published a report *Rights, Relationships and Recovery* (Scottish Executive, 2006) that set out a similar, though different, statement about the nature of mental health nursing within contemporary society. Each of the two reviews was developed through consultation with users of a wide range of mental health services, family carers, nurses and representatives of various professional health and social care bodies.

While nursing people with dementia occurs in different types of clinical areas by a range of nurses, it is mental health nurses who are usually involved in specialist dementia services. For this reason each of the two Reviews has considerable relevance for nursing people with dementia.

The key recommendations of *From Values to Action* that are relevant to mental health nurses working with people who have dementia are identified (see Insert 2:5).

Insert 2:5 Key messages from *From Values to Action* (DH, 2006)

- Mental health nursing should incorporate the broad principles of the recovery approach into every area of practice.
- All mental health nurses need to ensure that all groups in society receive an equitable service that reflects local population groups.
- Developing and sustaining positive therapeutic relationships with service users, their families and/or carers should form the basis of all care.
- Mental health nursing should take a holistic approach, seeing service users as whole people and taking into account their physical, psychological, social and spiritual needs.

Insert 2:5 cont'd

▶ Inpatient care should be improved though measures that include mental health nurses spending more time in direct client contact and minimising the time spent on administrative tasks.

▶ Mental health nurses need to be involved in risk assessment and management.

▶ Mental health nurses should focus on working directly with people of high levels of need and supporting other workers to meet less complex needs.

▶ Pre-registration training courses should be reviewed to ensure that essential competencies are gained at the point of registration and that relationships between service providers and higher education institutions should be strengthened.

▶ Career structures for mental health nurses should be reviewed according to local needs, and a range of new nursing roles should be developed and provided by provider organisations.

Rights, Relationships and Recovery (Scottish Executive, 2006)

The overall approach of *Rights, Relationships and Recovery* (Scottish Executive, 2006) is similar to that of *From Values to Action* (DH, 2006) and sets out its key messages accordingly (see Insert 2.6).

Insert 2:6 Key messages from *Rights, Relationships and Recovery* (Scottish Executive, 2006)

▶ Mental health nursing is focused on caring about people, about spending time with people, and on developing and maintaining helpful relationships with service users and their families and carers.

▶ We need to continue to develop rights-based and person-focused mental health care by promoting values and principles-based practice in mental health nursing.

▶ The recovery approach should be adopted as the model for mental health nursing care and intervention, particularly in supporting people with long-standing mental health problems.

▶ We need models of practice that are centred on relationships between mental health nurses and people, maximise nurses' contact time with service users, families and carers, and promote rights and recovery-based working.

Practice and services

▶ We need to support the development of mental health nurses' role in priority areas of acute inpatient, crisis care and intensive home treatment services.

▶ In particular we need to support and develop the role of the mental health nursing in acute inpatient care.

Insert 2:6 cont'd

- Mental health nursing will continue to have a key role in contributing to people with long-term and complex mental health problems and needs to adopt strengthens-based to working with people towards recovery.
- The role of mental health nursing in providing early intervention to people at risk of developing mental health problems needs to be developed and enhanced.
- Mental health nurses need to develop their role in relationship to health improvement, health promotion and in tackling inequalities.
- People who use mental health services want more access to 'taking therapies' such as psychosocial interventions and psychological therapies, but demand outweighs supply. We need to increase opportunities for mental health nurses to be developed to deliver these therapies.

Education and development

- We need to attract the right people into mental health nursing and make sure they are trained in the right way. A national framework that will ensure consistency of content and standards throughout Scotland is necessary to achieve this.
- All mental health nurses, whatever their area of work, need opportunities to continue to learn and develop.
- We need to actively involve service users, families, carers and practitioners in the design and delivery of education programmes for mental health nurses.
- We need to develop the role of health care support workers matching the skills and roles of health skills workers to people's needs.
- Leadership is the potential for realising the potential of mental health nursing for Scotland.
- We need to strengthen the capability for research and evaluation in mental health nursing.
- Build on existing developments and develop a learning community.

Making it happen

- Everyone needs to play their part in building strong alliances to bring about change.

While the focus of the two reviews is concerned with all areas of mental health nursing, they nevertheless provide ideas and guidelines that can be specifically applied to dementia care nursing. Of particular value is the way each review develops a value basis to mental health nursing that supports such important issues as maintaining dignity and ensuring the privacy of people with dementia. In addition, *Rights, Relationships and Recovery* (Scottish Executive, 2006) advocates the development of 'a whole-systems approach' that adopts a broad systemic approach towards mental health nursing which is similar to that put forward in *Everybody's Business* (DH, 2005a).

Of particular note is the reviews' support for 'the recovery approach' that asserts that the underlying rationale of mental health nursing is recovery. However, the idea of recovery does not fit well with nursing people who have a progressive and degenerative condition. While, *From Values to Action* (DH, 2006) claims that the recovery approach has 'successfully been used in services for people with severe dementia (p. 17)', it is unable to give any references to support this claim! At this point in time therefore, the idea of recovery is largely unexplored and untested within dementia care nursing and seems to draw more on nursing other client-groups within mental health care.

What Is Nursing People with Dementia?

At the beginning of this chapter, nursing people with dementia was described as a practical activity that is concerned with what nurses say and do. We believe that the distinctiveness of nursing lies its application of various theoretical frameworks, such as bio-medical and psychological frameworks to different clinical settings as a means of creating a care plan. Barker et al.'s (1997) definition of mental health nursing can be used to understand dementia care nursing and suggests that it:

- is an interactive human activity concerned with promoting the physical and psycho-social well-being of the person with dementia and their family members.
- includes physical activities that address the bodily care of the person with dementia; some nurse's work will involve areas of social taboo such as attending to people's elimination needs and other body fluids. Nurses working with people who have dementia should never be too posh to wash!
- is concerned with episodes of psychosocial distress arising from the onset and development of dementia.
- is associated with engaging in a mutually sustaining relationship through which subjective experience and social position is co-constructed.
- is linked to problems of everyday living that arise from having dementia and finding themselves increasingly out of step with social expectations. Nurses work alongside people with

dementia and their families as they co-navigate their shared journey through dementia.

We would want to augment this understanding of dementia care nursing through the addition of further concepts.

Well-being

The Department of Health document (DH, 2001) *Commissioning Framework for Health and Well-being* defines 'well-being' as 'The subjective state of being healthy, happy, contented, comfortable and satisfied with one's quality of life. It includes physical, material, social, emotional ('happiness'), and development and activity dimensions (p. 99). This definition is helpful though slightly confusing, as while it suggests that 'well-being' is a 'subjective state', it also includes physical and material dimensions. We also would identify physical and material dimensions of well-being and recognise the contribution made by purposeful activity. However, we would want to see well-being as not just a 'subjective state' but rather in holistic terms as relating to physical, psychological and social aspects of the personhood. In this way, people may have physical, psychological and social well-being and that all three are interrelated. We would also add that all people have the potential for well-being and this includes people with dementia, family carers and nurses, and the extent to which they possess and display well-being will affect other people's experience of it.

Reflection

Since the 1980s, nursing, including dementia care nursing, has been seen as a reflective practice (Jasper, 2004). Jasper succinctly defines 'reflective practice' as the 'means that we learn by thinking about things that have happened to us and seeing them in a different way, which enables us to take some kind of action (p. 2)'. In this way reflection upon people and situations may be seen as a way of gaining new knowledge within particular clinical situations and supports the legitimacy of evidence gained by reflection within dementia care nursing. However, we would want to take a rather more critical and systemic view of reflection and say first that nurses should reflect upon who occupies positions of power in particular clinical situations and how that power is used. We would suggest that often people with dementia find themselves quite powerless, and that nurses need to recognise and challenge these situations. People with dementia, family carer(s), other health and social care workers will have their own agenda which may be at odds with that of the person with dementia. This approach is adopted by Bolton (2005) who says that 'reflection'

> attempts to work out what happened, what they thought or felt about it, why, who was involved and when, and what these others might have experienced and thought and felt about it. It is looking at whole scenarios from as many angles as possible: relationships, situation, place, timing, chronology, causality, connection, and so on, to make situations and people more comprehensible. (p. 9)

Body

The importance of the body in nursing has been recognised by Lawler (1993) and more recently in mental heath care by Phillips (2006). A key idea within this present book is that people with dementia, family members and nurses all have bodies, and that 'the body' needs to be incorporated into any understanding of dementia care nursing. As Kontos (2005) urges, 'we must develop a new paradigm that respects individuals with Alzheimer's disease as embodied beings deserving dignity and worth (p. 565)'.

Acknowledging that the body is important in dementia care nursing because it is through the changes in the brain and other bodily organs that people experience dementia. Moreover, when a person with dementia is wet or in pain, it is through their body that it is experienced. As one person with dementia notes, 'When I trip over something, I get mad. I do believe that Alzheimer's does include what your feet do and what your hands do, as well as what your brain does (Henderson, 1998: p. 8).' In addition, it is through the body that nurses come into contact with people who have dementia and though which they assess and implement nursing care (Kontos, 2005).

The body also has a semiotic role and constitutes a collection of signs and messages that are displayed and read by the person with dementia, family members and the nurse. A person with dementia may show signs of tiredness by their bodily posture and facial expression that the nurse needs to read and address. 'Reading the body' is an important part of dementia care nursing, as many people with dementia often find it difficult to communicate through talk and can only make themselves understood through their body (Hubbard et al., 2002). But also the way nurses and carers use their body in relation to the person with dementia and the meanings that are made available have a significant impact upon the promotion of well-being. One particular situation occurs when nurses and carers need to touch intimate parts of the body, and in these situations they must ensure that the signs and messages that are available for the person with dementia to read promote their well-being.

Voice

People with dementia have views and opinions and there is a moral obligation upon nurses and family members to listen to what people with dementia are saying as they make their views and choices known. The idea of 'voice' used here has a more political connotation than is generally used in everyday speech. It is the voice of the less able person, in this case someone with a cognitive impairment, and is closely associated with not having power. Often people with dementia find that their views, interests and agendas are passed over and that those of other people, family members, medical practitioners, nurses and informal carers are given priority. Sometimes stories that are shared within dementia care situations represent people with dementia as not having the ability to say anything worthwhile; and so their voice is never heard and sometimes never sought. Thus people with dementia are often given no opportunity to make their views known, and have no opportunity to take part in decision-making processes such as those that occur between nurses and other health care professionals, and have no opportunity to make their views and opinions known. Because they are not allowed to have a voice, people with dementia often find themselves disempowered and subject to other people's wishes and agendas. There is thus a close relationship between voice and well-being as people who have a voice are more likely to find themselves included and possess dignity and well-being.

Story

Stories that arise and are shared between people with dementia, family members and nurses are particularly important within dementia care nursing, as they enable people to understand their own experience of having dementia or giving care and allow them to construct with others what has, what will and what may happen (Adams, 1999). Stories told by people with dementia and their carers have two related functions. First, they allow them to explore and articulate their own experience of having dementia or giving care and set it within a personal narrative that offers them a coherent, storied understanding of events. Second, stories contribute to the organisation of clinical settings by offering people different identities, responsibilities and obligations. One story may identify one person as attention-seeing, while another may identity them as needing care. Each story may be used at various points during case meetings, each achieving different things such as raising the concern of the nurse or perhaps gaining admission to much sought-after respite care.

Within this context, we would suggest that stories that are available and used within clinical settings contribute to the well-being of the person with dementia and their family members, though it is important to note whose stories are being told, who has the ability to tell them and who benefits from them being told. In this respect, people with dementia and, to a lesser extent, other family members are often at a disadvantage as their stories are not usually as universally recognised as are those of professionals and they themselves may lack the ability to share them convincingly, perhaps through their lack of cognitive ability or professional training.

Implicit in this view of 'story' is that there is often not just one dominant story that may be applied to a particular dementia care setting such as the story of a particular family member or the expert story of the doctor but rather that different stories may be mapped on to clinical settings, each giving a particular version of events. The Critical Realist position adopted in the book recognises the possibility of multiple of accounts or versions of events that can be 'mapped' on to situations (see Rolfe, 2000: pp. 42–45). No one story should therefore be seen 'the Truth' as each story arises out of a particular matrix of social relationships and advantages some people, while disadvantaging others.

Evidence

Alongside a growing recognition of the importance of voice and story, has been the increased recognition of evidence within nursing care (Rolfe, 2006). The view has arisen that research studies that largely occur outside practice areas, typically in university research sites, offer the strongest form of evidence and that the most cogent arises from randomised controlled trials (Sackett et al., 1996). We would take a wider and more inclusive view and argue that studies such as these are not the only source of evidence available to dementia care nurses and that other sources of evidence include:

- past experience – professionals seeing what works best with particular clients and/or personal experience taken from everyday experience of life situations;
- theory – such as Kitwood's person-centred care;
- views and opinions of people with dementia, family members and other health and social care workers;
- role models and experts;
- policy directives.

Thus, we see evidence in dementia care nursing as not merely contained in expert bodies of knowledge that are detached and separate from the clinical setting but rather as also including evidence that arises as people with dementia and their carers talk about situations. Indeed, within the whole systems approach outlined in this book, we would say that additional evidence comes from wider sources such as the media, culture and the government. But it is not just nurses who need evidence to make decisions, if decision-making is at all shared within dementia care, people with dementia and carers also need an evidential basis to their decision-making. We would also want to suggest that there is a close relationship between evidence and story and that evidence draws on culturally available accounts, stories and narratives such as the medical account of dementia, stories that are available about families and older people and accounts that are available about mental health care.

I remember working as a Community Mental Health Nurse in one town in the North of England in which the specialist dementia units were contained in part of the old workhouse that had always been known as 'Bottom Block'. Over the years, the older people I worked with had heard plenty of stories about people being sent to Bottom Block and what may have happened to them. These stories, *whether they were true or not*, affected how they saw mental health care in the town and my role in particular. Thus stories that arose and were shared between different people in the town contributed to decisions they made about the nursing care I was offering and were thus part of their evidence. Indeed, there is a sense in which all evidence are stories and that those stories that are used in decision-making as just those that are believed.

Summary

This chapter has introduced nursing people with dementia and initially examines its historical and socio-political context. The chapter describes the nature of nursing people with dementia and identifies key ideas that underpin its practice. Underlying this discussion is the view that nursing people with dementia is primarily a practical activity that nurses say and do and that it is guided and directed by theory. The chapter argues that nurses working with people who have dementia draw on different sources that offer evidence. These sources not only include evidence that is gained from research studies that have been undertaken outside the practice area, but includes evidence that arises during the course of conversational exchanges and social interaction within clinical settings. In this way, voice and story are important within dementia care nursing. In addition, the chapter asserts the importance of the 'body' and that not only is people's experience of dementia is physical and embodied but also that the body is an important way people with dementia receive care. The next chapter and the rest of the book develop these ideas and describe how nurses are able to promote the well-being of people who have dementia and their families.

References

Adams, T. (1999). Developing partnership in dementia care: a discursive model of practice. In T. Adams and C. Clarke (eds) *Dementia Care: Developing Partnerships in Practice*. Edinburgh: Baillière Tindall.

Barker, P., Reynolds, W. and Stevenson, C. (1997). The human science basis of psychiatric nursing theory and practice. *Journal of Advanced Nursing* 25, 660–667.

Berrios, G. E. and Freeman, H. L. (1990). Dementia before the twentieth century. In G. E. Berrios and H. L. Freeman (eds) *Alzheimer and Dementia*. London: Royal Society of Medicine Services Ltd., pp. 9–27.

Bolton, G. (2005). *Writing and Professional Development* (2nd ed.). London: Sage.

Butterworth T. (1998). Breaking the boundaries. *Nursing Times* 84, 47: 36–39.

Commission for Health Improvement (2003). *Investigations Arising from Care on Rowan Ward, Manchester Mental and Social Care Trust*, London: TSO.

Davies, S. (2003). Creating community: the basis for caring partnerships in nursing homes. In M. Nolan., G. Grant., J. Keady and U. Lundh (eds) *Partnerships in Family Care*. Maidenhead: Open University Press. pp. 218–237.

Department of Health (1994). *Working in Partnership: A collaborative Approach to Care*. Report of the Mental Review Team. London: HMSO.

Department of Health (1999). *National Service Framework for Mental Health*. London: Department of Health.

Department of Health (2001). *National Service Framework for Older People*. London: Department of Health.

Department of Health (2005a). *Everybody's Business. Integrated Mental Health Services for Older Adults: A Service Development Guide*. London: Care Services Improvement Partnership (CSIP).

Department of Health (2005b). *Securing Better Mental Health for Older Adults*. London: Department of Health.

Department of Health (2006). *From Values to Action*. London. Department of Health.

Gilliard, J., Means, R., Beattie, A. and Daker-White, G. (2005). Dementia care in England and the social model of disability. *Dementia: the International Journal of Social Research and Practice* 4, 4, 571–586.

Goffman, E. (1965). *Asylums*. Harmondsworth: Pelican

Greene, J. (1968). The psychiatric nurse in the community service. *International Journal of Nursing Studies* 5, 175–184.

Gunstone, S. and Robinson, J. (2007). The Right Route: service user involvement in care pathways. In J. Keady, C. Clarke, and S. Page *Partnerships in Community Mental Health Nursing and Dementia Care: Practice Perspectives*. Buckingham: Open University (in press).

Healthcare Commission (2006). *Living Well in Later Life: A Review of Progress against the National Service Framework for Older People*. London: Healthcare Commission.

Henderson, C. S. (1998). *Partial View: Alzheimer's Journal*. Dallas: Southern Methodist University Press.

Houliston, M. (1961). *The Practice of Mental Nursing*. Edinburgh: E. & S. Livingstone.

Hubbard, G., Cook, A., Tester, S. and Downs, M. (2002). Beyond words older people with dementia using and interpreting nonverbal behaviour. *Journal of Aging Studies* 16, 155–167.

Jasper, M. (2006). *Beginning Reflective Practice*. Cheltenham: Nelson Thornes.

Kitwood, T. (1997). *Dementia Reconsidered*. Buckingham: Open University Press.

Kontos, P. C. (2005). Embodied selfhood in Alzheimer's: re-thinking person-centred care. *Dementia: The International Journal of Social Research and Practice* 4, 4, 553–570.

Lawler, J. (1993). *Behind the Screen*. Edinburgh: Churchill Livingstone.

Miller, A. and Gwynne, G. (1972). *A Life Apart*. London: Tavistock.

Moriarty, J. (1999). Use of community and long-term care by people with dementia in the UK: a review of some issues in service provision and carer and user preferences. *Aging and Mental Health* 3, 4, 311–319.

Norberg, K-G., Asplung, Rasmusseen, B. Nordahl, G. and Sandman, P-O. (2001). How patients with dementia spend their time in a psychogeriatric unit. *Scandinavian Journal of Caring Science* 15, 215–221.

Phillips, L. (2006). *Mental Illness and the Body: Beyond Diagnosis*. Routledge: London.

Repper, J., Brooker, C. and Repper, D. (1995). Serious mental health problems: policy changes. *Nursing Times* 91, 25, 29–31.

Robb, B. (1967). *Sans Everything*. London: Nelson.

Rolfe, G. (2000). *Research, Truth Authority: Postmodern Perspectives on Nursing*. Basingstoke: Macmillan.

Rolfe, G. (2006). Evidence-based practice. In M. Jasper (ed.) *Professional Development, Reflection and Decision-making*. Oxford: Blackwell Publishing, pp. 135–153

Sackett, D., Rosenberg, W., Gray, J., Haynes, R. and Richardson, W. (1996). Evidence-based medicine: what is it and what it isn't. *British Journal of Medicine* 312, 71–72.

Scottish Executive (2006). *Rights, Relationships and Recovery*. Edinburgh.

Department of Health (2005). *Securing Better Mental Health for Older Adults*. HMSO: London.

Sheldon, J. H. (1948). *The Social Medicine of Old Age*. London: Oxford University Press.

Chapter 3

People's experience of having dementia

Trevor Adams

Learning Outcomes

After reading the chapter you will be able to

- identify the shortcomings of the biomedical approach towards dementia;
- critically discuss person-centred approaches towards people with dementia;
- discuss the implications of person-centred approaches upon nursing practice;
- discuss the contribution of attachment to understanding people with dementia;
- outline the typical subjective experiences of people with dementia;
- evaluate how people's experience of dementia is socially constructed.

Introduction

This chapter describes different ways of thinking about what it is like to have dementia. These approaches may be applied to different clinical situations and are able to guide and direct how nurses should work with people who have dementia and their families. The chapter challenges exclusively biomedical approaches towards people with dementia that result in the institutionalisation, de-personalisation and marginalisation of people with dementia. As discussed previously, there are various shortcomings with bio-medical approaches towards dementia care, not least that they only represent the contribution of physical and biomedical phenomena. This chapter outlines alternative psycho-social approaches that provide insights into the ways well-being of people with dementia may be promoted.

Person-centred Dementia Care

Various psycho-social approaches towards people with dementia emerged in the first part of the twentieth century (Gilhooly, 1984). These approaches had little impact on nursing, and as we saw in Chapter 2 an institutional approach towards people with dementia prevailed. During the 1970s, however, various psychological approaches were introduced into mental health care for older people such as Reality Orientation and Reminiscence Therapy that offered new ways of viewing and thinking about people with dementia and addressed the long-standing therapeutic nihilism within dementia care (Lyman, 1989).

By far the most influential of these approaches was person-centred care. This approach developed in the late 1980s through the work of Tom Kitwood at the University of Bradford, United Kingdom (see Downs, 2000; Brooker, 2006). The primary innovation of person-centred care was to redirect attention from biomedical aspects of dementia to the subjective experience of people with dementia. This led to people with dementia, particularly in the early stages of the condition, being seen as able to make sense of their situation, as having feelings, and as possessing value, worth and dignity.

Kitwood's initial argument was that professional practice towards people with dementia had been underpinned by the bio-medical approach. Kitwood argues that within the medical profession there existed a 'hypothesis of exclusive neurological causation' (Kitwood, 1987b) which claimed that the behaviour of people with dementia was entirely due to neuropathological processes. Kitwood challenges this view and argues that people's experience of dementia arises out of a dialectical relationship between physical health/ neurological impairment and social/psychological factors.

'Personhood' is a central idea in person-centred care which Kitwood defines as 'a standing or a status that is bestowed on one human being, by another in the context of relationship and social being' (Kitwood, 1997: p. 8). In addition, Kitwood sees personhood as transcendent, sacred and unique; and that it accords people who have dementia with an ethical status that offers them absolute value resulting in an obligation 'to treat each other with deep respect' (Kitwood, 1997: p. 8).

Kitwood links personhood with the provision of care and describes different interactive processes that may occur in dementia care settings that impair personhood. He calls these processes 'malignant social psychology' and sees them as having a malign effect on personhood and contributing to the development of dementia. Kitwood describes 17 'malignant social psychologies'. One type of malignant social psychology is 'treachery'. This occurs when different forms of deception are used to manipulate or gain control over a person with dementia. This may happen when a nurse says something that is untrue to a person with dementia so that they can get them to do something they would not otherwise do. When this occurs, the person with dementia feels betrayed and humiliated (just like you would!), and contributes to their downward decline into dementia.

Another malignant social psychology Kitwood identified is 'objectification'. This occurs when a person with dementia is treated as if they had no opinions or feelings, just like dead matter. This may happen in many situations such as when a nurse removes someone's clothes without noticing that they can be seen by other people or when a nurse is talking to another nurse about what they were doing the previous night without any thought that the person with dementia is beside them. All these forms of interaction would have a malignant effect on anyone's personhood, but even more so, with someone who has dementia.

Kitwood argues that the progression of dementia is not necessarily downward and that through good communication, which he calls 'positive person work', a person's condition may improve and lead to 'rementia'. Kitwood (1997) outlines ten different forms of 'positive person work'. One form of positive person work is recognition. This occurs when a person acknowledges that a person with dementia is a person. Nurses may do this by speaking to someone with dementia by *their* preferred name, by affirming their views or simply by thanking them for what they have done. Another form of positive person work is play. This occurs when people with dementia are enjoying themselves by doing activities that engender spontaneity, self-expression and fun.

Recent Developments within Person-centred Care

There have been two recent important developments within person-centred care. Each of these developments displays a faithfulness to Kitwood's original work but shows signs of extending his original approach.

The first formulation may be seen in the work of Brooker (2006) and her development of the equation:

Person-centred care $= V + I + P + S$,

in which,

V = a value base that asserts the absolute value of all human lives regardless of age or cognitive ability,

I = an individualised approach, recognising uniqueness,

P = understanding the world from the perspective of the service users,

S = providing a social environment that supports psychological needs.

Brooker's reformation of person-centred care is useful and enables more recent ideas such as citizenship and social inclusion to be integrated into person-centred care.

The second reformulation is displayed in the recent work of the *Center for Research on Personhood in Dementia* based at the University of British Columbia (O'Connor, 2007) and is concerned with moving beyond 'the immediate interactional environment' (p. 133) and recognises 'positioning the dementia experience within a broader context. Context may be conceptualised as including, for example, race and ethnicity, social location, organisational practices and policies, and social discourses' (p. 133). While the contribution of broader social context formed part of Kitwood's early writing on dementia care, it soon fell out of view. This second reformulation of person-centred care is certainly welcome and anticipates an increased recognition of the contribution of social, cultural and political domains within whole systems approaches towards dementia care that are more fully discussed in Chapter 6.

Shortcomings of Kitwood's Person-centred Care

Although Kitwood's ideas are attractive, various shortcomings have been identified in his approach to person-centred care (see Adams, 1996; Harding and Palfrey, 1997; Parker, 2001; Epp, 2003; Davies, 2004; Adams, 2005). The first shortcoming is concerned with serious methodological flaws that are contained in Kitwood's empirical research. While most of Kitwood's writings on dementia care are theoretical, from time to time he refers to his own important early research. This work involved compiling over 44 'psycho-biographies of people with dementia that outline significant life events and describing how these events have contributed to the person's dementia' (Kitwood, 1993). However, the validity of these psycho-biographies is seriously impaired because they are compiled from interview data containing the views of relatives rather than the person with dementia. In addition, Kitwood adopted a rather naïve approach to language that assumes that what was said by carers was always what had happened. But people do not always 'tell it as it is' and often put their own view on what has happened. Kitwood's study of psychobiographies was never reviewed by his peers and subsequently published, as is the custom within the scientific community. The only peer-reviewed paper that arose from Kitwood's study was taken from one psycho-biography taken from data given by the relatives of a woman called Rose (Kitwood, 1990).

A further shortcoming of person-centred care is that while Kitwood's underlying dialectical approach highlights the contribution of physical/neurological impairment *and* social/psychological phenomena to the dementia process, much of Kitwood's writing only seems to highlight social and psychological processes and does not give similar attention to the contribution of ageing and pathological processes. The psycho-social focus in Kitwood's work should be seen against the backdrop of 1970s and 1980s, when there was a need to challenge the dominance of the medical approach and its contribution towards institutionalisation and de-personalisation. While Kitwood's focus on social and psychological aspects of dementia is perfectly understandable in its wider historical context, his work now seems polarised and increasingly out of date. Recent developments relating to the diagnosis of dementia, new pharmaco-logical treatments (Adams and Page, 2000) and genetics (Schutte and Holston, 2006) have led to a need to reaffirm Kitwood's recognition of the dialectical relationship between bodily/pathological and social/psychological processes in people with dementia. While this more balanced view of dementia exists in Kitwood's initial work, in his later work it tended to be overshadowed by the contribution of psycho-social phenomena.

A different view is now beginning to emerge and, indeed, Downs et al. (2006) reassert the dialectical approach initially developed by Kitwood and identify it with the bio-psycho-social model of health, developed by the World Health Organisation (WHO, 2002). In addition, this approach is supported in empirical studies. Surr (2006), for example, highlights the relationship between embodi-ment, interaction and the sense of self in people with dementia;

Phinney and Chesla (2003) show that bodily and somatic phenomena are commonly experienced by people with dementia; and Kontos (2006) develops the idea of 'embodied selfhood'. This latter idea argues that the body is an active and communicative agent that is imbued with its own wisdom, intentionality and purposefulness, and is separate and distinct from cognition. 'Embodied selfhood' is a new and important idea that not only offers nurses a fuller understanding of people's lived experience of dementia but also allows people with dementia to be seen as able to express themselves through their body (Kontos, 2006).

A similar idea is found in the work of the philosopher Margaret Archer (2000) who argues that people's sense of self arises as a result of the 'primacy of practice', through their action. In relation to the 'primacy of practice' she argues that 'One of the most important properties that we have, the power to know ourselves to be the same being over time, depends upon practice in the environment rather than conversation in society' (p. 7). Thus, unlike Kitwood, who argues that people's sense of identity arises from what other people say to them, Archer (2000) argues that people primarily gain a sense of self by what they say and do with their bodies; that is their practice. We would incorporate Archer's proactive and embodied understanding of selfhood into our understanding of people with dementia and suggest that personhood arises not only, as Kitwood says through other people's actions, *but also* through what people with dementia say and do themselves. Archer's understanding of selfhood is important for nurses, as it supports the participation of people with dementia in purposeful activities as a means of promoting their well-being.

Regarding personhood as merely arising through social interaction is highly problematic as it implies that people with dementia are only people when others acknowledge and talk to them. An extreme version of this approach may support the views of Dworkin (1993), who has asserted that 'Demented people in the late stages of the disease have lost the capacity to recognise, appreciate or suffer indignity' and that 'It is expensive, tedious and difficult to keep seriously demented patients clean, to assure them space for privacy, to give them the personal attention they often crave' (p. 234). If personhood merely arises through social interaction and ideas, such as those of Dworkin, become more widely accepted and perhaps come to influence government policy, people with dementia may find themselves being given fewer rights than other people and not being regarded as really human.

A third shortcoming of Kitwood's work is concerned with the way informal carers are represented within person-centred care. Some have pointed out that person-centred care leads to the family being blamed for the progression of the dementia. Davis (2004) comments that 'Even the kind and well-intentioned carer may directly affect the disabling process' and argues that in person-centred care ' ... if a carer feels that the person they had a relationship with exists no more, then they themselves are directly involved in the dissolution of personhood' (p. 376). Other people have seen person-centred care as a rather narrow approach that highlights the person with dementia at the expense of the rest of the family. Nolan et al. (2002) argue that person-centred care fails to 'capture the interdependencies and reciprocities that underpin caring relationships' (p. 203) and suggest that person-centred care does not fully represent the 'mutual appreciation of each other's knowledge, recognition of its equal worth, and its sharing in a symbolic way to enhance and facilitate joint understanding' (Nolan et al., 2002: p. 204).

The last shortcoming is that within person-centred care interaction between informal/formal carers and people with dementia is typically seen as unidirectional and concerned with how informal and formal carers communicate *to* the person with dementia. Brooker (p. 219) claims that person-centred care takes place within the 'context of relationships'. However, this is misleading as Kitwood does not think of people with dementia as primarily initiating verbal interaction with other people. We would therefore challenge Kitwood's view of communication within dementia care and argue that people with dementia are not merely the recipients of other people's interaction but rather can initiate interaction themselves and that communication is not unidirectional but a two-way street (Haak, 2003).

Before leaving the idea of person-centred care, it should be noted that within health and social policy a different understanding of person-centred care has developed. Standard Two of the *National Service Framework for Older People* (DH, 2001), for example, is concerned with person-centred care and asserts that it occurs when 'NHS and social care services treat older people as individuals and enable them to make choices about their own care' (p. 23). However, the *NSF for Older People* (DH, 2001) has a broader understanding of person-centredness that incorporates the individualisation of care to the user and the informal carer. As Brooker notes 'The way to achieve person-centred care is by listening to the views of users and carers about the services they need and want, and this is strongly promoted within the NSF' (p. 23) and argues that this is a 'far cry' (p. 21) from Kitwood's understanding of 'person-centred care'.

Moreover, *Dementia: supporting people with dementia and their carers in health and social care: NICE Clinical Guide* (NICE/CSPI: p. 6) puts forward 'the importance of relationships and interactions with others to the person with dementia, and their potential for promoting well-being' as an underpinning principle of person-centred care and asserts the importance of considering 'the needs of carers, whether family and friends or paid care workers, and to consider ways of supporting and enhancing their input to the person with dementia' (p. 6). In this way, person-centred care as it is viewed in recent health and social care policy is much nearer to how it is understood in the whole systems approach adopted in this book (see Chapter 6) rather than in Kitwood's person-centred care.

Hearing the Voice of People with Dementia

One implication of person-centred care is that people with dementia should be viewed as able to talk and sometimes write about what it is like to have dementia and the type of services they would like to receive. This approach commends nurses to 'hear the voice of the person with dementia' and argues that just because someone has dementia does not mean that they are incapable of having views and opinions of their own. Indeed, a growing body of empirical research has found that people with dementia often do have a voice (Feinberg and Whitlatch, 2000). Good practice is therefore concerned with making every effort to hear and listen to the voice of people with dementia.

Numerous people have written about their experience of having dementia (Davis, 1989; McGowin, 1993; Bryden, 2005). Froggatt's early work found that while the cognitive self may be affected by memory loss, the experiencing/feeling self may be less impaired and that people with dementia may possess self-awareness (Froggatt, 1988: p. 133). This idea allows the possibility that even though a person's memory may be impaired, positive therapeutic engagement may still occur through such means as positive person work and the use of different healing arts.

This idea was extended by Cottrell and Schulz (1993) who highlighted that the views and opinions of people with dementia were hardly ever heard in research studies. More recently, various methods of hearing the voice of the person with dementia have been put forward and used within research studies (Wilkinson, 2002). The implications of hearing the voice of people with dementia and their carers in research are discussed by Clarke and Keady (2002), and an increasing number of studies now include the participation of people with dementia.

Goldsmith's work had a seminal effect within dementia care and initiated many people's awareness of the voice of people with dementia. In his book *Hearing the Voice of People with Dementia: Opportunities and Obstacles* (Goldsmith, 1996), Goldsmith identifies recent trends in social policy that promote the increased involvement of users within service provision and argues that this provides opportunities for people with dementia. Goldsmith asserts that communication with people who have dementia is possible and suggests that it is because people with dementia are not allowed to speak out that they resort to measures that are often seen by professionals and family carers as 'challenging and problem behaviours'. Goldsmith commends professionals to listen to what people with dementia are trying to say and asserts that professionals are often in too much haste and do not give people with dementia enough time to say what they want. In addition, Goldsmith argues that the interior design of many care settings often prevents good communication and that it should promote the ability of people with dementia to express their views.

A similar approach is advocated by Barnett (2000), who argues that people with dementia are part of the feedback loop with service provision and that to evaluate whether a particular service has been effective it is important and necessary to seek the views of people with dementia. Barnett says that people with dementia are often treated as 'non-persons' and are not seen and treated as full members of society. As well as exploring issues associated with the effectiveness of service towards people with dementia, Barnett argues that hearing the voice of the person with dementia has a positive effect on everyone involved in the provision of care and enables staff to gain worthwhile insights about the provision of care.

This view of 'voice' is developed more fully by Procter (2001) in her study about listening to older women with dementia. Procter argues that there is an alternative, non-dominant view of 'the order of things' to which people with dementia are giving voice. This view may challenge the views of many nurses and family carers, but nevertheless constitutes the view of the person with dementia. This understanding of voice raises issues about different and possibly competing 'truths' that exist in dementia care settings and supports the argument that dementia care nurses should listen to different voices, not least the voice of the person with dementia.

Attachment Theory and People with Dementia

A further approach that offers worthwhile insights into people's experience of dementia is outlined by Miesen and Jones (1992). Their work seeks to explain the emotional world of people with dementia by applying various psychological theories such as Bowlby's attachment theory (Bowlby, 1980) and reminiscence theory (Coleman, 2005). Miesen and Jones (1992) develop the idea of 'patient orientation' in which people with dementia think that one or both their parents are still alive when in fact they have been dead for a few years.

Underlying this approach is the idea that babies and young children form attachments to one or more figures and that separation from these figures leads to psychological distress in their absence and pleasure when they return. Moreover, at times of stress, for example, when they are in a 'strange situation' they are likely to seek out an attachment figure and gain psychological support from their presence. The child's attempt to find an attachment figure is described as 'attachment behaviour'. Empirical evidence suggests that attachment security remains a key feature of people's relationships through their life and will affect their ability to secure relationships and emotional stability (Bowlby and Bowlby, 2005).

With regard to people with dementia, Miesen (1992, 1995) found that they develop 'an awareness context' and have some awareness of the seriousness of their condition. For them, being forgetful and confused is 'a strange place'. Miesen shows that there is a strong relationship between the extent of a person's parent fixation, their cognitive functioning and displaying displacement behaviours such as asking how their parents are, calling out and searching for their parents and begging to go to their parental home. Miesen argues that the reduced ability of people with dementia to retain information leads to them feeling unsafe and experiencing a strange situation. In these situations, their awareness context declines from a more or less permanent state to one that is temporary or momentary and so they become 'a displaced person' (Miesen and Jones, 1997).

Miesen's approach is attractive and is supported by established psychological theory. It offers a theoretical basis upon which dementia care nurses can underpin nursing care plans aimed at reducing a person's disturbed behaviour through the sensitive use of communication. Most of all, the approach challenges the idea that people with dementia are deliberately difficult or aggressive and offers an explanation why many become agitated and emotionally disturbed (Browne and Slosberg, 2006).

Keady and the Early Experience of People with Alzheimer's Disease

Keady (1999) in a study of in-depth interviews with primary family carers to people with dementia identified the following stages associated with informal caregiving.

Slipping
The first stage is 'slipping' and occurs when a person in the early stages of dementia starts to be aware of minor and trivial slips and lapses in memory and/or behaviour. These slips are initially ignored, but as they become more frequent, they can no longer be dismissed. At this stage 'emotion-focused coping' (see Chapter 2) such as 'discounting' or 'normalising of events' is often used to dismiss the significance of events.

Suspecting
Slipping gradually fades into 'suspecting'. As episodes of forgetfulness occur with increasing frequency or severity, they can no longer be rationalised or ignored. Attempts to minimise the significance of these episodes through 'discounting' or 'normalising of events' become less successful as coping strategies and the person begins to suspect that something could be quite seriously wrong.

Covering up
During this period, the person with dementia makes a conscious and deliberate effort to compensate for difficulties that are occurring and actively hides them from family members, friends and colleagues. As the dementia progresses, covering up becomes more difficult and the person with dementia begins to restrict activities in certain areas where it is difficult to maintain competence. If family members have not done so already, they may now begin to notice changes in the level of cognitive and behavioural activities.

Revealing
During this period, the person with dementia reveals their difficulties to their closest friends and relatives. This may be due to a conscious decision or the result of being confronted by patterns of loss. At this stage, knowledge about the emerging difficulties may be kept within the immediate family and formal confirmation of suspicions may be delayed.

Confirming
Open acknowledgement about the presenting difficulties is made and the process of diagnostic confirmation may begin.

Maximising
The person continues to adjust to having dementia through the use of adaptive coping techniques to compensate for accumulating losses.

Disorganisation
Cognitive and linked behavioural problems experienced by the person with dementia become an increasingly dominant feature. They may display a diminishing ability to make decisions and a loss of awareness of actions.

Decline
Normal and overtly reciprocal relationships become clouded and uncertain. The instrumental demands of care become a prominent feature of caregiving relationships, together with an increased dependency. At some point during this period, the person with dementia may need to leave their home and enter into continuing care.

Death
The person will dementia enters the last phase of their life. During this period, they will need palliative care. Eventually, however, their life will end.

Keady later refined this model and provided more detail about the first six stages that is from 'slipping' to 'maximising'. In this later revision, Keady argued that people with dementia enter into a period of transition that involves adaptive coping strategies. These strategies were accompanied by the person with dementia experiencing fear, anxiety and great uncertainty. Keady identifies two interdependent strategies that are encountered by people with dementia: 'taking stock' and 'sharing the load'.

Taking stock is preceded by an awareness and self-acknowledgement that something is wrong. The first signs of occurance may include problem-solving difficulties, lack of concentration, word-finding problems, labile emotions, feeling and becoming lost in once familiar surroundings, writing block and decline in co-ordination and control of speech and actions. Keady and Gilliard (1999) found that these signs usually were not ascribed to Alzheimer's disease but rather were seen as nuisances and sometimes as an embarrassment and a sign that things were not right.

'Taking stock' comprises three tactics.

Closing down

The primary purpose of 'closing down' is to allow time to adjust to the new-found reality and to re-frame existing events. This is a self-protective strategy aimed at maintaining the person's integrity and their sense of who they are. 'Closing down' was expressed by the following set of coping strategies:

- keeping real feelings and fears secret;
- withdrawing from conversations;
- remaining in familiar surroundings;
- constantly repeating things to oneself to aid memory;
- weeping when no one is around;
- keeping as active as possible;
- trying to avoid new situations as far as possible;
- relying on oneself to solve problems.

Re-grouping

This is a time-limited tactic aimed at providing the person with the confidence and resilience to 'keep going'. This tactic involves an acceptance of the purpose of 'closing down' and an acceptance that reality cannot return to normal. This tactic draws on a range of coping strategies that include self-belief and draws on the familiarity of someone's surroundings and on support from family and friends. Keady and Gilliard (1999) describe how people with Alzheimer's disease use this tactic to talk to themselves as a means of gaining confidence for the future.

Covering your tracks

This describes the tactic used by the person with as yet, undiagnosed Alzheimer's disease so that their condition will not be found out. This tactic may also be shared with the close family members and gives rise to the condition being a secret within the family. However, initially covering your tracks is used to retain control over the individual's situation and to continue the tacit collusion. The person with dementia may employ various coping strategies to control the progress of the undiagnosed Alzheimer's disease. These strategies include

- keeping fears and feelings secret;
- using lists and other memory aids;
- constantly repeating things to oneself to help with memory problems;
- keeping further memory loss to oneself for as long as possible;
- fighting memory loss so it will not 'get the better of you';
- engaging in mentally challenging activities such as puzzles and crosswords;
- making up stories to fill the gaps;
- trying to remain calm at all times;
- taking things one day at a time.

Owing to the secretive nature of this tactic, people with Alzheimer's disease often experience some lowering of mood during this period. Covering your tracks is associated with the investment of 'physical and emotional energy' and thus the somatic nature of the strategy may be seen. The tactic of 'covering your tracks' often continues for some time. It often becomes quite difficult for family members to collude unwittingly with events that occur; concealment becomes difficult and breaks down.

Sharing the load

This period is characterised by unburdening oneself and may be associated with a number of options and possibilities. It may occur as family members decide to confront openly their relative with dementia or more subversively seek the independent opinion of the General Practitioner. Sometimes the person with (undisclosed) Alzheimer's disease may decide to disclose their experiences to a friend or a close family member. 'Sharing the load' is a cathartic experience and an opportunity to get things out into the open. Coping behaviours that occurred at this time included

- being thankful for the close support of family members and other people;

- relying on the support of the person who is closest to you;
- trying to keep relaxed at all times;
- talking about one's memory loss to people.

It should be noted though that sharing the load may not be total and concealment may still occur at this stage. Sharing the load has implications for the involvement of nurses as there is a responsibility to support people with dementia and family members who have been told the diagnosis. Sharing the diagnosis is often very difficult for health care professionals; as the Audit Commission (2000) showed, many people with dementia are never told that they have dementia. However, Keady and Gilliard (1999) note that the provision of a diagnosis helped people with dementia put what was happening into context and allowed them to give friends and family members an explanation.

Social Disability and Dementia

Some recent theorists have put forward a social disability model of dementia (Adams and Bartlett, 2003; Gilliard et al., 2005). This model offers a radical understanding of dementia that views people with dementia as having a disability and argues that services have used medical categories to define people and their limitations rather than their strengths and abilities. Through these means the social disability approach argues that people with dementia are negatively represented in society and frequently find themselves disadvantaged and excluded. Some supporters of this approach claim that this process feeds the 'disability industry' and makes people with disabilities 'victims'. Barnes (2003) has suggested that the essence of the social model of disability 'represents nothing more complicated than a focus on economic, environmental and cultural barriers encountered by people viewed by others as having some form of impairment' (p. 9). Gilliard et al. (2005) believes that this definition corresponds well with people's experience of what it is like to have dementia.

The disability approach is associated with the idea of 'excess disability' that describes the discrepancy between a person's impairment and what is warranted by their functional incapacity (Brody, 1971). For example, a person may be blind but the effect of the condition is increased by how they are treated by other people. Sabat (2001) applies the idea of excess disability to people with dementia and argues that malignant social psychology leads to 'excess disability'.

People who argue that dementia is a social disability view people's experience of dementia as being similar to the experience of people who have other disabilities such as impaired sight or hearing. While there are many similarities between the social disability model of dementia and Kitwood's person-centred care, we would argue that the social disability model offers nurses a more comprehensive understanding of the contribution of socio-political phenomena to people's experience of dementia.

When applied to nursing people with dementia, the social disability model would support approaches that

- increase the participation of people with dementia within the design and development of services;
- increase the use of non-medical language to describe what people can do;
- continue 'normal' activities that allow the person with dementia to be seen as 'ordinary' in the best sense of the word
- listening to the 'voice' of people with dementia particularly when decisions are being made that will affect them;
- allow people with dementia to have equal access to rationed services.

We see all these interventions promoting the well-being of people with dementia.

The Social Construction of Dementia

There are two main approaches towards social construction (Danziger, 1997). The first is called the 'strong programme'. This is a top-down approach that is concerned with how issues in society such as sexuality, crime and mental health are constructed by different 'discourses' that shape people's views of the world and themselves. Harding and Palfrey (1997) apply this approach to dementia care and describe how discourses lead to normalisation and surveillance. The second approach is called the 'weak programme' (the term does not imply that it is a poor programme!). This programme describes micro-social and interactive processes in society that lead to how people and situations are constructed and represented in everyday social situations. Various elements of this weak form of social constructionism may be seen in the work of Kitwood (1997) and Sabat (2001).

Sabat (2001) focuses on how interactive episodes lead to the construction of identity in people with Alzheimer's disease. Sabat argues that the way language is used, particularly in relation to words that relate to selfhood, gives rise to the way people with dementia view themselves. Sabat (2006) outlines three forms of self:

Self 1: This form of self refers to the 'self of personal identity' and is experienced when a person with dementia uses first person indexicals such as 'I', 'me', my' and 'mine'. When a person with dementia uses the word 'I' in the sentence 'I want to go home,' they are locating themselves as an 'I' in the social world and showing others that they are the source of that wish. The use made of pronouns by the person with dementia allows them to be seen as having a Self 1, and also allows them to experience that self. Underpinning this view is the idea that language not only just represents the world but also constructs it and constructs people's experience of themselves.

Self 2: This represents the self of physical and mental attributes, past and present. These would include a person's religious, political and social beliefs, and personal qualities like their particular sense of humour, as well as what they think about having these characteristics. A person will lose some of these aspects of Self 2 as a result of having dementia – for example, a person with dementia will lose many of the skills they may have acquired at university, however, other aspects of self will be retained, for example they will still be a university graduate. In addition, they will gain new aspects of Self 2, for example, they will always be a university graduate.

Self 3: Refers to the self of multiplicity of social personnae, which does not reflect a single unified self, but a multiplicity of selves. For example, a person may have different personal identities: they may be a father, a nurse and a churchgoer. This manifestation of Self 3 in social contexts cannot be accomplished without the help of others. Therefore, the identities that constitute Self 3 are the result of conversational exchanges and are co-constructed as the person with dementia talks with other people.

Sabat (2006) illustrates this understanding of the tripartite self and its construction within dementia care through a number of case studies that illustrate that while people with Alzheimer's disease (AD) may report the striking loss of some cognitive abilities various forms of selfhood that exist within Self 1, Self 2 and Self 3 still remain. Sabat argues that these forms of selfhood are not diminished as a result of the disease, but rather through 'the lack of cooperation given by others' (Sabat, 2006: p. 337).

Sabat's work is helpful as it helps nurses understand how they and family members may be responsible, in part, for diminishing the selfhood of people with dementia. Sabat's work bears many similarities to Kitwood's, though Sabat does not adopt a dialectical approach and does not recognise the bodily and embodied experience of people with dementia.

The work of Harding and Palfrey (1997) adopts the strong programme towards social constructionism and examines the contribution of wider social processes to the construction of people with dementia and their care.

Underpinning their work is the idea that particular people come to be identified as having dementia through expert knowledge that is created and made available by the medical profession. They argue that 'dementia or Alzheimer's disease is an example of a socially constructed disease, and the major players in such a construction – its architects as it were – are the medical profession' (p. 4). The medical profession thus defines what constitutes normal behaviour in society and differentiates it from abnormal behaviour. Thus, anyone whose behaviour does not conform to what society expects may find themselves identified as having dementia and being treated in a way that is made acceptable by the medical profession.

Harding and Palfrey (1997) draw on Foucault's understanding of the body and gaze in which he argues that twentieth-century society has been redefined and resembles an organic system, a body whose cells comprise its human members. So where once illness was seen to affect human cells, it is now seen to affect social spaces and relationships that lie between people. In this way, people and their relationship with family members and friends are made visible and society comes under the full gaze of the medical profession.

Harding and Palfrey (1997) point out that when society is seen as a body then those that are not in full health – the old and the infirm – are seen as deleterious to the whole body. Within this context, people with dementia are seen as being unable to exert self-control and so pose a possible threat to the social body in much the same way as cancer threatens the physical body. In these circumstances 'the demented' need to be controlled, and as institutional care is too costly, social control through community care needs to be developed.

The examination of relationships in society and the identification that one of its members might have dementia is accomplished by various agencies including general practitioners and the primary health care team; checks for people over the age of 75 years may be seen as one way in which this may occur (Trickey et al., 2000). More specifically, the work of memory clinics may be seen as one way in which the medical profession identifies new cases of dementia in society and organises social relationships to address its demands.

This approach has much in common with the work of Gilleard and Higgs (2000) who drew on Elias' idea of the civilising process. With respect to people with dementia, Gilleard and Higgs (2000) argue that 'A body [which] the mind has lost control of becomes instead the de-civilized body' (Gilleard and Higgs, 2000: p. 168). Moreover, they describe the way the State has extended its role and now occupies a civilising role within society. This role constructs informal agencies such as family members as regulating and controlling people who are de-civilised as a result of dementia. Within this context, Gilleard and Higgs (2000) elaborate on how recent approaches such as the construction of assessment tools and the development of 'person-centred care' has increased the ability of the State to exert control over older people, ensure regulation and maintain the orderliness of society.

The work of Harding and Palfrey (1997) and Gilleard and Higgs (2000), therefore, views people's experience of dementia as socially and politically constructed and enables nurses to see how nursing might be part of a broader, societal approach towards older people. In addition, the approach provides insights into particular ways that older people may be understood as 'confused' that may lead to their marginalisation and exclusion within society. Insights such as these are important because they enable nurses to recognise how they may contribute to this process and that what they say and do may give rise to people with dementia not being included within dementia care. The insights offered by this approach help nurses develop care plans that promote inclusion of the person with dementia within decision-making processes.

Summary

This chapter has looked at different psychological and social approaches towards people with dementia. These approaches go beyond narrow biomedical approaches that view people with dementia as little more than bodies. The approaches outlined recognise that the cognition of people with dementia largely remains in tact long after onset and that emotional feelings continue irrespective of people's cognitive impairment. While people like Dworkin (1993) have argued that people with dementia do not share the 'humanness' and 'personhood' as other people, we would suggest that

Summary cont'd

these approaches allow people with dementia to be seen as possessing the same rights and expectations as other people (McIntyre, 2003).

Despite the important contribution made by different psychological and social approaches towards dementia, many of them have shortcomings, as they tend to focus on the person with dementia and offer few insights into other people associated with the dementia care setting. This is a serious omission as research has consistently shown that relatives and nurses frequently contribute to people's experience of having dementia and also incur physical and emotional distress as they live and work alongside people with dementia (see Adams and Manthorpe 2003). The physical and emotional labour of looking after someone with dementia is discussed more fully in Chapter 10. We would, however, support many of the ideas contained in approaches that primarily focus only on the person with dementia but rather than seeing these approaches as the only approach that may be used in dementia care nursing would see them as offering one part of a much wider picture that not only includes the person with dementia but also other members of the family, local health and social care, private and voluntary agencies and government policy relating to older people with dementia. We understand this as a whole systems approach.

References

Adams, T. (1996). Kitwood's approach to dementia and dementia care: a critical but appreciative review. *Journal of Advanced Nursing* 23, 948–953.

Adams, T. (2005). From person-centred care to relationship centred care. *Generations Review* 15, 1, 4–7.

Adams, T. and Page, S. (2000). New pharmacological treatments for Alzheimer's disease: implications for dementia care nursing. *Journal of Advanced Nursing* 31, 1183–1188.

Adams, T. and Bartlett, R. (2003). Constructing dementia. In T. Adams and J. Manthorpe (eds) *Dementia Care*. London: Arnold. pp. 3–21.

Adams, T. and Manthorpe, J. (2003) *Dementia Care*. London: Arnold.

Archer, M. (2000). *Being Human: The Problem of Agency*. Cambridge: Cambridge University Press.

Audit Commission (2000). *Forget Me Not: Mental Health Services for Older People*. London: Audit Commission.

Barnes (2003). What a difference a decade makes. Reflections on doing 'emancipatory' disability research. *Disability and Society* 18, 1, 3–18.

Barnett, E. (2000). *Including the person with dementia in designing and delivering care.* London: Jessica Kingsley.

Bowlby, J. (1980). *Attachment and Loss. Loss, Sadness and Depression.* London: Hogarth Press.

Bowlby, J. and Bowlby, R. (2005). *The Making and Breaking of Affectional Bonds.* London: Routledge.

Brody, E. (1971). Excess disability of mentally impaired aged. Impact of individualised treatment. The *Gerontologist* 225, 124–133.

Brooker, D. (2006). *Person Centred Care.* London: Jessica Kingsley.

Browne, C. J. and Slosberg, E. (2006) Attachment theory, ageing and dementia: a review of the literature. *Ageing and Mental Health* 10, 2, 134–142.

Bryden, C. (2005). *Dancing with Dementia.* London: Jessica Kingsley.

Clarke, C. L. and Keady, J. (2002). Getting down to brass tacks: a discussion of data collection with people with dementia. In H. Wilkinson (ed.) *The Perspectives of People with Dementia: Research Methods with Motivations.* London: Jessica Kingsley, pp. 25–46.

Coleman, P. (2005). Reminiscence: developmental, social and clinical perspectives. In M. L. Johnson, (ed.) The *Cambridge Handbook of Age and Ageing*, Cambridge: Cambridge University Press, pp. 301–315.

Cottrell, V. and Schulz, R. (1993). The perspective of the person with Alzheimer's disease: a neglected dimension of dementia research. *Gerontologist* 33, 2, 205–11.

Danziger, K. (1997). The varieties of social construction. *Theory and Psychology* 7, 3, 399–416.

Davis, D. H. J. (2004). Dementia: sociological and philosophical constructions. *Social Science and Medicine* 58, 2, 369–378.

Davis, R. (1989). *My Journey into Alzheimer's Disease.* Amersham: Scripture Press.

Department of Health (2001). *The National Service Framework for Older People.* London: DH.

Downs, M. (2000). Dementia in a socio-political context: an idea whose time has come. *Ageing and Society* 20, 3, 369–375.

Downs, M., Clare, L. and Mackenzie, J. (2006). Understandings of dementia: explanatory models and their implications for the person with dementia and therapeutic effort. In J. C. Hughes, S. J. Louw and S. R. Sabat (eds), *Dementia: Mind, Meaning, and the Person.* Oxford: Oxford University Press, pp. 235–258.

Dworkin, R. (1993) *Life's Dominion.* New York: Knopt.

Epp, T. D. (2003). Person-centred dementia care: a vision to be refined. *Canadian Alzheimer Disease Review*. April 14–18.

Feinberg, L. F. and Whitlatch, C. J. (2001). Are persons with cognitive impairment able to state consistent choices? *The Gerontologist* 41, 3, 374–382.

Froggatt, A. (1988). *Self-Awareness in Early Dementia*. In B. Gearing, M. Johnson and T. Heller (eds) *Mental Health Problems in Old Age*. Buckingham: Open University Press.

Gilhooly, M. L. M. (1984). The social dimensions of senile dementia. In I. Hanley and J. Hodge (ed.) *Psychological approaches to the care of the elderly*, pp. 88–135.

Gilleard, C. and Higgs, P. (2000). *Cultures of Ageing: Self, Citizen and the Body*. Harlow: Prentice Hall.

Gilliard, J., Means., R. Beattie, A. and Daker-White, G. (2005). Dementia care in England and the social model of disability. *Dementia* 4, 4, 571–586.

Gillies, B. A. (2000). A memory like clockwork: accounts of living through dementia. *Aging and Mental Health* 4, 4, 366–374.

Goldsmith, M. (1996). *Hearing the Voice of People with Dementia: Opportunities and Obstacles*. London: Jessica Kingsley.

Haak, N. J. (2003). "Do you hear what I mean?" A lived experience of disrupted communication in mid-to-late stage Alzheimer's disease. *Alzheimer's Care Quarterly* January/March 2003, pp. 26–39.

Hamilton, H. E. (1994). *Conversations with an Alzheimer's Patient: An Interactional Sociolinguistic Study*. Cambridge: Cambridge University Press.

Harding, N. and Palfrey, C. (1997). *The Social Construction of Dementia: Confused Professionals*. London: Jessica Kingsley.

Jones, G. M. M. and Miesen, B. M. L. (eds) (1992). *Care-giving in Dementia: Research and Applications*. Volume 1. London: Tavistock/Routledge.

Keady, J. (1999). *The Dynamics of Dementia: A Modified Grounded Theory Study*. PhD Thesis, Bangor: University of Wales.

Keady, J. and Gilliard, J. (1999). The early experience of Alzheimer's disease: implications for partnership and practice. *Dementia Care: developing partnerships in practice*. Edinburgh: Ballière Tindal. pp. 227–256.

Kitwood, T. (1987). Dementia and its pathology: In brain, mind or society? *Free Associations* 8, 81–93.

Kitwood, T. (1990). Understanding senile dementia: a psychobiographical approach. *Free Associations* 19, 60–76.

Kitwood, T. (1993). Towards the reconstruction of an organic mental disorder. In A. Ridley (ed.) *Worlds of Illness: Biographical and Cultural Perspectives on Health and Disease*. London: Routledge, pp. 143–160.

Kitwood, T. (1997). *Dementia Reconsidered*. Buckingham: Open University Press.

Kontos, P. C. (2006). Embodied selfhood: the expression of ethnographic of Alzheimer's disease. In A. Leibing and L. Cohen (eds), *Thinking about Dementia: Culture, Loss and the Anthropology of Senility*. New Brunswick: Rutgers University Press, pp. 195–217.

Lyman, K. A. (1989). Bringing the social back in: a critique of the biomedicalisation of dementia. *The Gerontologist* 29, 5, 597–605.

McGowin, D. F. (1993). *Living in the Labyrinth: a Personal Journal Through the Maze of Alzheimer's*. Cambridge: Mainsail Press.

McIntyre, M. (2003). Dignity in dementia: person-centred care in the community. *Journal of Aging Studies* 17, 473–484.

Miesen, B. M. L. (1992). Attachment in dementia. Bound from birth? In G. M. M. Jones and B. M. L. Miesen (eds), *Care-giving in Dementia: Research and Applications*. London: Tavistock/Routledge, pp. 103–132.

Miesen, B. M. L. (2006). Attachment theory and dementia. In G. M. M. Jones and B. M. L. Miesen (eds), *Care-giving in Dementia: Research and Applications*. Volume 4. London: Tavistock/Routledge, pp. 38–56.

NICE/CSPI (2006). *Practice Guide NICE/SCIE: Dementia: Supporting People with Dementia and their Carers in Health and Social Care: NICE Clinical Guide 42*. London: NICE/CSPI.

Nolan, M., Ryan, T., Enderby, P. and Reid, D. (2002). Towards a more inclusive vision of dementia care practice. *Dementia: The International Journal of Social Research and Practice* 1, 2, 193–211.

Nolan, M. R., Davies, S., Brown J., Keady, J. and Nolan J. (2004). Beyond 'person-centred' care: a new vision for gerontological nursing. *Journal of Clinical Nursing* 13, s1, 45–53.

O'Connor, D., Phinney, A., Smith, A., Small, J., Purves, B., Perry, J., Drance, E., Donnelly, M., Chaudhury, H. and Beattie, L. (2007). Personhood in dementia care: developing a research agenda for broadening the vision. *Dementia* 6, 1, pp. 121–142.

Parker, J. (2001) Interrogating person-centred dementia care in social work and social care practice. *Journal of Social Work* 1, 3, 329–345.

Phinney, A. and Chesla, C. A. (2003). The lived body in dementia. *Journal of Aging Studies* 17, 285–299.

Procter, G. (2001). Listening to older women with dementia. *Disability and Society* 16, 3, 361–376.

Sabat, S. (2001). *The Experience of Alzheimer's Disease: Life Through a Tangled Veil.* Oxford: Blackwell.

Sabat, S. (2006). The self in dementia. In M. L. Johnson (ed.), *The Cambridge Handbook of Ageing.* Cambridge: Cambridge University Press, pp. 332–337.

Schutte, D. L. and Holston, E. C. (2006). Chronic dementing conditions, genomics, and new opportunities for Nursing Interventions. *Journal of Nursing Studies* 38, 4, 328–334.

Scottish Executive (2006). *Rights, Relationships and Recovery.* Edinburgh: Scottish Executive.

Surr, C. A. (2006). Preservation of self in people with dementia living in residential care: a social-biographical approach. *Social Science and Medicine* 62, 1720–1730.

Trickey, H., Turton, P., Harvey, I., Wilcock, G. and Sharpe, D. (2000). Dementia and the over 75 check: the role of the primary care nurse. *Health and Social Care in the Community* 8, 1, 9–16.

Wilkinson, H. (ed.) (2002). *The Perspectives of People with Dementia: Research Methods and Motivations.* London: Jessica Kingsley.

World Health Organisation (2002). *Towards a Common Language for Functioning, Disability and Health.* London: World Health Organization.

Chapter 4

Dementia: understanding the neurological contribution as a basis to nursing practice

Elizabeth Anderson

Learning Outcomes

After reading the chapter you will be able to

- identify the contribution of biological phenomena to personhood;
- describe the contribution of different aspects of the brain to the development of dementia particularly with respect to people's language and behaviour;
- discuss how understanding the contribution of biomedical phenomena may help nurses communicate with people who have dementia;
- discuss how nurses need to take full account of the limitations placed on the person with dementia by biological aspects of dementia.

Introduction

In Chapter 1, we argued that dementia arises from a dialectical process through which biomedical and social/psychological factors mutually contribute to people's experience of dementia. The purpose of this chapter is to review current knowledge about the nature of the neurological impairment in dementia in order to ground the understanding of what it means to have the condition at the biological level. This knowledge is necessary to get the balance between biomedical and social/psychological factors right and to clearly articulate the relationship between neurological aspects of dementia and those that arise as a basic result of people's social and psychological setting. By adding this neurological understanding to Kitwood's understanding of the dialectics of dementia, the contribution of bio-medical factors may be clarified and will enhance the understanding of nurses working with people who have dementia.

What is Dementia?

The World Health Organisation (2003) has recently defined 'dementia' as

> A syndrome due to disease of the brain, usually of a chronic or progres-sive nature, in which there is disturbance of multiple higher cortical functions, including memory, thinking, orientation, comprehension, cal-culation, learning capacity, language and judgement. Consciousness is not clouded. The impairments of cognitive function are commonly accompanied, and occasionally preceded, by deterioration in emotional control, social behaviour or motivation. This syndrome occurs in Alzheimer's disease, in cerebrovascular disease, and in other conditions primarily or secondarily affecting the brain.

This chapter examines the neurological changes that occur in dementia and highlights the implications they have for people with dementia and their nursing care. It is hoped that these insights will help nurses enhance the well-being of people with dementia and make a positive contribution towards their care. The WHO defin-ition identifies the core feature of dementia as the 'disturbance of [the] multiple higher cortical functions' of the brain. The word 'cortical' makes reference to the cortex, a vast sheet of nerve cells that covers the whole surface of the brain. The cortex is an important control centre between sensory information coming into the brain and motor commands leaving the brain. Complex networks of cells within the cortex are dedicated to processing sensory information to a very high level, resulting in high-level cognitive skills such as conscious perception, thought, language, memory, planning and decision-making.

The emergence of these complex functions depends upon cooperation between different areas of the cortex that have become specialised for different purposes. Within the cortex there is a hierarchy of primary, secondary and association areas (see Figure 4.1; the primary and secondary areas are shaded and the association areas are unshaded). Primary areas are closest to sensation or action; that is, they are either the first point of call for

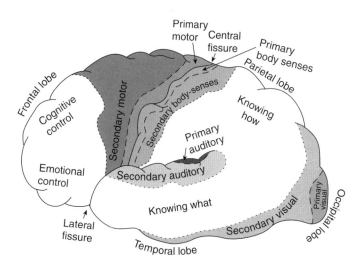

Figure 4.1   Simplified scheme of the basic functional divisions of the cerebral cortex

sensory information coming into the cortex or the last point of call for motor commands leaving the cortex. There are three distinct areas of primary sensory cortex, one for the three main sources of incoming sensory information (the ears, the eyes, and the body). Primary motor cortex exists as a single area and is the last point of call for outgoing commands to the body for action. Figure 4.1 shows that the three areas of primary sensory cortex are behind the central fissure (a deep cleft that divides the cortical sheet into a back and a front section), whilst the primary motor cortex is in front of the central fissure. This highlights an important point about cortical organisation: the cortex behind the central fissure deals with sensation and understanding, whilst the cortex in front of the central fissure deals with action and behaviour (Luria, 1973).

Secondary cortex is one level removed from sensation or action. In the case of sensation, secondary sensory cortex learns patterns, through experience of the external world, that impose order on the raw sensory information logged in the primary areas. These patterns form sensory representations that are the perceptual basis for the recognition of things, for example, the recognition of certain visual stimuli as objects of people or of certain auditory stimuli as words. Secondary motor areas perform a similar function for action. They learn patterns that tie together the sub-components of skilled actions. Take, for example, the complex series of body movements required for speaking a word. This intricate coordination of throat, mouth, tongue and chest movements occurs efficiently and accurately because of learnt patterns in secondary motor cortex that tie the component movements together into 'motor representations' for the required act.

The sensory and motor representations within the secondary networks are advanced and complex but they are limited to their specific sensory domain or to the control of actions. In the secondary network there is no integration of information across the senses or between sensory and motor functions. Integration occurs at the highest level of the cortical hierarchy, in the areas of association cortex. This integration of information across the senses results in a higher level of awareness and the rich, multi-faceted and abstract knowledge of the world that is unique to humans.

Primary (organic) dementia occurs when the highest areas of the cortex, that is the association parts of the cortex, get disrupted by brain damage. This may be a result of direct damage to the cortex (for example, as in Alzheimer's disease or cortical Lewy body disease) or indirect disruption through damage to the subcortical structures that support and regulate cortical activity (for example, as in subcortical vascular dementia or Parkinson's disease). Secondary (functional) dementia occurs when the functions of the association cortex are disrupted by causes that do not directly damage the brain but disrupt its processing powers (for example, depression, nutritional deficiency or hypothyroidism). Because secondary dementias do not directly damage the brain, these forms of dementia are usually reversible, and the dementia is not a long-term condition for those affected. The purpose of this chapter is to draw out the care implications for those who have irreversible dementia. Thus, for the remainder of this chapter the focus will be on primary dementia, using Alzheimer's disease as the prototype with caveats drawn for other primary causes where necessary.

Alzheimer's disease is the most common cause of primary dementia and it is now known that this disease does not damage the brain randomly, but specifically targets cells in the association areas of the cortex, leaving the primary and secondary areas relatively unharmed until the disease becomes very advanced (Pearson et al., 1985; Lewis et al., 1987). The preservation of the dedicated primary and secondary regions of both sensory and motor cortex means that the person continues to log and perceive incoming sensory information and retains the basic capacity for purposeful action. However, the damage to the knowledge structures of the association areas, which make sense of that information and allow it to influence behaviour, are increasingly impaired. Thus, as Alzheimer's disease develops, the person's understanding of what is seen, heard and felt becomes increasingly fragile and the world becomes increasingly unfamiliar and uninterpreted.

Problems with Knowledge: 'Knowing What' and 'Knowing How'

In the sensory cortex, the association areas behind the central fissure are fundamental to the emergence of knowledge about what people see and do. Knowledge divides into two main types: 'knowing what' knowledge, which is the domain of the temporal association areas, and 'knowing how' knowledge, which is the domain of the parietal association areas (Goodale et al., 1993; see Figure 4.1). 'Knowing what' refers to the ability to have high-level knowledge about things that are seen, heard or felt, whilst 'knowing how' refers to the spatial knowledge that mediates skilled inter-action with what is seen, heard or felt. If you consider a mug, 'knowing what' knowledge refers to the ability to know that it is a receptacle for hot drinks, whilst 'knowing how' knowledge refers to the ability to pick up a mug and drink from it. Because these two types of knowledge are represented separately it is common for people with primary dementia, particularly in the early stages, to have damage to one type of knowledge but not the other. Thus, it is common to find people with dementia who can use a mug but not know what it is, or who know what it is but cannot use it.

Language and 'Knowing What'

'Knowing what' knowledge is strongly associated with language. The majority of the brain exists within two halves called the cerebral hemispheres. Thus, the cortex is also divided; one half of the sheet covers the surface of the left hemisphere, whilst the other half covers the surface of the right hemisphere. In most people, language functions are located predominantly in the left hemisphere and thus language problems typically indicate damage to this side of the brain. Within the left hemisphere language is made possible by complex communications between the primary and secondary areas dedicated to sensory and motor functions, and the temporal association areas that provide the interpretative 'knowing what' knowledge base (sometimes called 'semantic memory'). In primary dementia, particularly Alzheimer's disease, language difficulties are usually associated with damage at the knowledge level. Thus, although people with Alzheimer's disease are often said to be aphasic, that is, they have a language disorder, the language problems are usually an aspect of a more central agnosia, that is, a knowledge disorder. The sparing of the primary and secondary areas of the cortex means that the sensory and motor aspects of language often remain intact, at least during the mild to moderate stages. The person remains able to hear speech and to speak, but the understanding that allows them to understand either what is said or what they say is increasingly compromised (Martin and Fedio, 1983; Murdoch et al., 1987). Some people with Alzheimer's disease can read out text loud quite fluently but are unable to understand what they are reading (Bayles et al., 1991; Lamdon-Ralph et al., 1995). Other forms of primary dementia, such as vascular dementia, strike the cortex more randomly and may damage the sensory and motor aspects of language function rather than, or in addition to, the knowledge aspects. Thus, a person may have an intact knowledge base but have a specific difficulty either with understanding the speech of others or with speaking coherently themselves. It is important, therefore, to observe and assess a language disorder in a person with dementia carefully.

Returning to Alzheimer's disease, the first sign of the deterioration of the 'knowing what' knowledge base is anomia, that is, the inability to name objects or to find words in conversation. However, as the disease develops the consequences become more pervasive, undermining not only knowledge of what words mean but also of what objects and faces mean (Hodges et al., 1992, 1993). The failure to recognise people, even close members of the family, is a symptom that can cause particular distress to relatives. It is important that relatives understand that this symptom is a consequence of neurological impairment and does not indicate that the person with dementia does not care for them or value them. The attention of relatives should be orientated, instead, towards whether or not the person is pleased to see them. Murdoch et al. (1987) found that people with Alzheimer's disease were able to make correct judgements about the pleasantness or unpleasantness of words they could not understand. It is important to know that the consciously accessible part of knowledge represents but the tip of an iceberg built upon foundations that extend deep into subconscious processes, both within the cortex itself and in the many subcortical structures that lie beneath. Thus, when interacting and communicating with people who have dementia, nurses need to remember that whilst the conscious access to knowledge may be disturbed, the underlying foundations that direct action and emotion may remain intact. Body language, and other non-verbal signals such as facial expression and tone of voice, provide an access route to these deeper foundations, providing an alternative means of communication when language is compromised.

'Knowing How' and Visuo-spatial Functions

The temporal association areas have been characterised as being essential for 'knowing what' knowledge. The parietal association areas, by contrast, are essential for 'knowing how' knowledge (see Figure 4.1). 'Knowing how' knowledge is not mediated by words and description but by the ability to coordinate and skilfully control the body in response to visual information. Damage to the parietal association areas results in apraxia, an impairment of skilled movement despite normal sensory and motor capabilities.

The right parietal lobe is important for appreciating space and for directing attention across space. This is likely to show up as constructional apraxia, an inability to understand how parts fit together into a spatially organised whole. Driving ability is severely undermined by damage to this part of the cortex which, as an area of association cortex, is vulnerable to Alzheimer's disease and other organic causes. Most people who get primary dementia develop problems with spatial cognition at some point in the course of their illness and have to relinquish their driving licences. This can cause conflict between people with dementia who want to maintain their independence and families and paid-for carers who recognise the serious risk of driving without spatial cognition. Problems with drawing and copying also arise (the copying of the pentagon figure in the MMSE tests this function) as well as problems in controlling objects in space (for example, in guiding cutlery to the dinner plate) or being able to work out how clothes fit onto the body (dressing apraxia). Wandering, where people want to walk but become lost and disorientated even in familiar surroundings, is another common symptom associated with damage to the parietal lobe (de Leon et al., 1984) although the desire to walk is natural and the walking behaviour itself should not necessarily be seen as a symptom of dementia, but rather as a 'symptom' of being human; for advice on understanding the psychosocial context of wandering see Stokes, 2002.

Damage to the left parietal lobe is associated with visuo-spatial difficulties relating to language and mathematical functions. The parietal association area of the left hemisphere is an important nexus in the flow of information required for 'the 3 Rs', reading, (w)riting and 'rithmatic. These abilities are usually affected in primary dementia. Once spatial cognition is affected, mathematical ability is vulnerable because the understanding of number emerges from the understanding of space. The 'mental workspace' used for both mental arithmetic and logical reasoning depends upon these left-hemisphere parietal networks (Luria, 1973). Difficulties with 'mental workspace' abilities are common early in the course of dementia, although in the early stages of Alzheimer's disease this probably reflects the breakdown of neural communications within the cortex as a whole rather than direct damage to the parietal association area, the direct damage occurring later and intensifying the problem.

Helpful Responses to the Breakdown of Knowledge in Dementia

Alzheimer's disease usually causes bilateral damage to the temporal and parietal association areas of the cortex ultimately leading to significant disruption to 'knowing what' and 'knowing how' knowledge. As the disease develops, however, there is variation from one person to the next in terms of the balance of damage between the left and right hemispheres, and between the temporal and parietal lobes. Thus, especially in the earlier stages, symptoms do differ from one person to the next (Haxby et al., 1985; Martin, 1987). The outdated conceptualisation of dementia as 'global intellectual decline' can give rise to the belief that once someone has dementia the intellect sinks as an undifferentiated whole. However, it is not only possible but also likely that in each individual some abilities will be more severely affected than others because of differences in the underlying degree of damage to different areas of the cortex. Thus, there is no justification to believe that, because someone can do one thing but not another, they must have given up and are simply not trying any longer with the impaired ability.

Furthermore, it was noted earlier that knowledge rests on deep foundations and that disruption at the highest level does not indicate that the whole knowledge structure has disappeared or failed. Dementia erodes knowledge slowly and there are things that can be done to help people with dementia make the most of the knowledge that remains. When cells begin to be stripped out of these knowledge networks the finer-grained aspects of knowledge get lost first, but many of the deeper structures remain intact. So, for example, word-finding difficulty for rare words, like 'trellis', precedes word-finding difficulty for common words like 'dog'. Or, a person may look at a hammer and know its category, a tool, but not its exact identity, a hammer (Martin and Fedio, 1983; Hodges et al., 1992). The ability to distinguish between two objects also depends upon how similar they are to one another; the greater the similarity the lower the chance of success. In a video about the neurological underpinnings of the dementia syndrome, the Dementia Services Information and Development Centre (2003) provides a good example in Jim, who is struggling to distinguish between a tube of toothpaste and a can of shaving foam. His inability to distinguish results in him smearing toothpaste on his face and receives an understandable response of consternation and disbelief from his wife. However, the deterioration of 'knowing what' knowledge explains why this action is not as silly as it seems. Furthermore, had Jim been making a choice between shaving foam and a mug he would probably have made the right choice. There are clear lessons that nurses may draw from this example; first, in not making rash judgements about what is silly, and second, in keeping environments simple and uncluttered. These are straightforward considerations that nurses can use to significantly help people with dementia to make the right choices, although in seeking to minimise clutter it is important not to go to the extreme and cause sensory deprivation instead.

Within the knowledge networks, knowledge does not exist within particular nerve cells, but rather in the pattern of activation across hundreds of thousands, perhaps even millions, of nerve cells. The ability of the association cortex to fulfil its function of making sense of sensory information depends upon a stable pattern forming within these vast networks of cells. The brain damage underlying primary dementia destabilises these networks, thereby reducing the chances of the activity settling into a recognisable pattern. As neural damage accumulates knowledge becomes at first unreliable and later inaccessible. However, there are many external factors that affect the signal-noise ratio in these networks and, therefore, the chances of stable patterns forming. In essence, anything that increases the noise reduces the chances of association cortex being able to make sense of the input. As Powell (2000) points out, talking whilst rushing around or over the top of the television sends a very noisy signal to the person's brain and is likely to result in the person not understanding. Similarly, anything that increases the strength of the key message, for example, by speaking clearly, simply and literally, maximises the chances of success. Nurses can help to prepare people with dementia by telling them the general topic of what they are going to talk about. This helps by activating information from memory that semi-prepares the patterns in advance.

Strengthening the signal through repetition or providing multiple sensory routes to the required knowledge also helps. Thus, it is helpful if nurses give the person the object being talked about or point to it. The use of mime and gesture is also valuable. Patterns need time to form, so giving the person additional time to understand is fundamental. Impatience will instigate anxiety in the person with dementia. This has the opposite effect, effectively sending 'neural shock waves' through the cortex and disrupting whatever patterns are trying to form. Checking glasses and hearing aids is also essential to ensuring that the quality of the incoming sensory information is optimal.

These techniques, recommended by Powell (2000), are aimed at improving communication and enhancing 'knowing what' knowledge, but the basic mechanisms of 'knowing how' knowledge are the same, and similar approaches are recommended for helping people with apraxia. Helping a person struggling with dressing apraxia by demonstrating the correct sequence so that they can copy, giving simultaneous verbal instruction to boost the strength of the signal and maybe sensitively touching appropriate body parts to orientate attention, can help a person to succeed (Dementia Services Information and Development Centre, 2003). Furthermore, even though knowledge is deteriorating it is important to keep activating what remains; the less often the patterns are instantiated the more quickly they will become unattainable.

Problems Associated with Damage to the Frontal Association Cortex

The previous discussion has covered the 'knowing what' and 'knowing how' functions of the temporal and parietal association areas behind the central fissure. In this section, the functions of the association cortex in front of the central fissure, dedicated to the control of action and behaviour, will be discussed. These vast areas of frontal association cortex (quite exceptionally large in our species relative even to other primates) are responsible for translating knowledge into action and for making our behaviour voluntary and flexible, driven internally by what we want to do rather externally by habits or instincts stimulated by the environment (Luria, 1973).

The upper regions of the frontal association cortex are primarily concerned with the integration of cognitive information into the decision-making process to make behaviour efficient with respect to current goals (see the area labelled 'cognitive control' in Figure 4.1). Damage to this area results in stereotyped, habitual and inefficient behaviours (Luria, 1973). So, for example, if a person sees a door they may be compelled by habit to try and open it and continue to keep trying despite the fact that it is locked, leading to escalating frustration. This is because the control mechanisms that signal failure and the need to stop or try a different tack have been undermined. Many institutions have found that painting doors with scenes to disguise them is helpful in preventing such behaviours. It is always important to consider how the environment may be impacting on the person by stimulating habitual behaviours that can no longer be controlled. Equally, explaining the situation is unlikely to be of help because the mechanisms that incorporate knowledge into the decision-making process are no longer working optimally. Again, the Dementia Services Information and Development Centre (2003) provides a good example of a lady laying the table one piece of cutlery at a time, rather than thinking ahead and taking all the cutlery required in one go. When the inefficiency of the strategy is explained by her daughter, the lady acknowledges this, but continues as before. Good relations between mother and daughter depend upon the daughter understanding that it is brain damage, and not a desire to be obtuse, that is causing her mother to ignore her good advice.

The lower regions of the frontal association cortex, by contrast, are primarily concerned with the integration of emotional information into the process, and in particular social rules concerning how we should manage our emotions and instincts (Damasio, 1994); see the area labelled 'emotional control' in Figure 4.1. Damage to this area causes little alteration to intellectual capabilities but is associated with profound personality changes. Overall, behaviour ceases to be controlled according to the needs of others or the long-term needs of the self. 'Me-now' becomes the only motivating force. Thus, symptoms relating to the breakdown of emotional and social behaviour can be associated with damage to this part of the frontal lobe (Damasio, 1994).

Having said this, however, extreme caution is needed in moving from the occurrence of emotional and social symptoms to the conclusion that the frontal lobe is damaged. Knowledge of the 'civilising' functions of the lower frontal lobe means that there is a particular danger that all changes in personality and behaviour are attributed to underlying damage to this region. The only form of dementia strongly associated with severe and early damage to this region is frontotemporal dementia, a relatively rare form of dementia that tends to affect people in late middle-age rather than in old age (Neary and Snowden, 2003). More common causes of dementia, such as Alzheimer's disease and vascular dementia, are not associated with a focus of damage in this area of the brain, particularly when the dementia is mild to moderate in severity. It is important to appreciate that the behavioural consequences of damage to the lower frontal lobe are intense and extreme. The behavioural symptoms more usually seen in dementia are more likely to be a normal reaction to the cognitive impairment, to the changes in everyday activity and social interactions that occur in response to the impairment or to the failure of other people to understand what the person with dementia is experiencing. In other words, such 'symptoms' are more likely to reflect an increase in provocations towards emotional distress, rather than a failure of the brain to control emotional processing.

Indeed, memory loss, the cardinal symptom of dementia, does not just have the obvious effect of forgetting appointments, shopping and so forth, but fundamentally alters the person's internal reality and belief system. Ongoing experience is increasingly understood in terms of the past owing to the greater resilience of old memories relative to the new. As damage to the memory system accumulates it becomes impossible for the person to keep up to date with change or to appreciate that their understanding of the world is departing from reality. From the perspective of people without dementia this departure is obvious, but people without dementia need to remember that although the brain of the person with dementia is damaged it nonetheless remains active and is in charge of their behaviour. The overall purpose of the brain is to make a person an active agent in managing behaviour and maintaining well-being. If, in the attempt to care for people with dementia their status as active agents is ignored and they are forced into situations that, from their perspective, threaten their independence and well-being, then they will respond actively to try to protect themselves from these changes. This issue of the relationship between a person's memory loss and the impact of other people's behaviour in response to that memory loss will be explored further in the next section focusing on memory impairments (for a more detailed account of what it might be like to live in the internal world of a person with dementia, see Stokes, 2000).

Problems with Memory and the Impact on Behaviour

Memory symptoms are at the core of the dementia syndrome and are also amongst the most complex to understand because memory involves intricate communications between a structure buried deep in the temporal lobe, called the hippocampus, the whole of the cortex and many other structures far beyond the scope of this review. Thus, there are multiple reasons for why the memory system may be disrupted in dementia. However, this review will again focus primarily on Alzheimer's disease, which causes direct damage to the hippocampus.

The hippocampus is essential for the instant, one-off learning that leads to rich memories of our experiences. This form of memory is sometimes called 'episodic memory' to contrast it with 'semantic memory' (which we have been calling 'knowing what' knowledge). The mechanisms by which episodic memory is made possible are very complex but, in essence, the cortex sends highly processed information into the hippocampus, and the hippocampal networks then tie the pattern of activation together into a memory unit. If the unit is later re-activated the hippocampus sends activation back out into the cortex, so that the pattern is re-created or replayed through the cortical networks, causing a muted re-experience of the original.

Damage to the hippocampus causes amnesia, a deficit in the ability to form consciously accessible memories of ongoing experience.

If significant numbers of nerve cells in the hippocampus are damaged then new memories become impossible and the person cannot remember anything that happened more than a few minutes ago. However, memories from long ago tend not to be affected because important memories are often replayed through the hippocampus– cortex feedback system, causing representations to form within the 'knowing what' networks of the temporal association cortex. Thus, in the early days of Alzheimer's disease, when the disease is confined to the hippocampal system (Braak and Braak, 1991), the person cannot remember new information but retains information about events from long ago. However, as we have already seen, the progressive nature of Alzheimer's disease means that it spreads out from the hippocampus to affect the 'knowing what' areas as well. At this stage the old memories also begin to fade, with the strongest and most familiar being the last to go.

As damage accumulates within the hippocampus and the 'knowing what' networks, the person's consciousness becomes increasingly dominated by strong memories from the past because the present can no longer get a foothold. At first glance, many beliefs and behaviours of people with dementia seem bizarre and unconnected with the present, but looking a little deeper it is usually the case that the beliefs and behaviours of people with dementia are related to what is going on now. So, for example, it is not that unreasonable for people with dementia to think that their grandchildren are their children. Family resemblance means that the face of a grandchild is likely to stimulate old memories about the child. However, damage to the hippocampus and temporal lobe prevents this fine distinction between the perception of the grandchild today and the memory of the child 30 years ago. Perhaps what is important is not that the relative is correctly identified but that both grandchild and child stimulate feelings of closeness and security and contribute to the person's sense of belonging and well-being. As was said earlier, fond memories and well-loved people and objects remain able to activate feelings of happiness, security and well-being long after the finer-grained factual detail has faded away because of the deep foundations of knowledge.

The other side of this coin, however, is that bad memories and threat-related people/objects can activate subcortical structures which have evolved to coordinate powerful anger and fear behaviours in response to threatening stimuli. When people with dementia manifest anxiety or aggression, it is important to be alert to the triggers and to determine whether these responses may be mediated by things or people in the environment. It is worth remembering that the ward or residential home is an unfamiliar environment full of unfamiliar people, strange activity and equipment and that the brain processes unfamiliarity as a form of threat. The relative invulnerability of many subcortical structures and also the primary and secondary 'feeling areas' (part of body-senses; see Figure 4.1) of the cortex means that people with dementia continue to engage in emotional behaviour, and to experience the associated feelings, both positive and negative, even though they increasingly do not understand why they may be doing or feeling those things. Thus, there is a duty of care upon all nurses to protect the person with dementia from ill-being and to promote the experience of well-being. Arguments that people with dementia are not capable of feeling pain or pleasure are not valid.

The behaviour of people with dementia also needs to be interpreted within the context of their life history because habits tend to be robust against cortical damage. A case study by a student described a man who had the strange habit of continually stroking and picking at the carpet in his room. This behaviour caused concern until it was discovered that the man used to be a carpet fitter. The behaviour gave the man a sense of occupation and thus was consequently seen as being helpful rather than deviant, considerably reducing conflict between staff and the man. This illustrates how the brain is fundamentally shaped by experience and indicates the importance of understanding behaviour in the context of the person and their past.

Furthermore, although the weakening of the networks within the hippocampus and temporal association cortex means that the beliefs of people with dementia become increasingly outdated, this does not weaken the force of their beliefs. From the person's perspective their beliefs apply today as much as they did in the past. Furthermore, these beliefs are feeding forward into the frontal mechanisms that control decision-making, and also down into subcortical structures that govern powerful survival behaviours and instincts. Thus, beliefs are not passive mental representations but are very active mental representations that motivate and guide behaviour. To understand the behaviour of people with dementia it is critical for nurses to 'tune in' to the world of the person and identify the beliefs that are motivating them.

Violet, for example, has dementia and is in residential care. It is dinner time but Violet does not want to come for dinner. Instead, she is frantically walking down the corridor saying that she must find 'Our Mary.' When the staff approach Violet and ask her to come for dinner she gets angry and shakes them off so that she can continue her search. At face value Violet's behaviour seems odd and unhelpful. However, during most of her life Violet has been a mother and a homemaker. Violet's brain has, therefore, generated lots of useful habits revolving around the organisation and care of children. Any mother knows that trying to get children out of the house on time is difficult and frustrating. It is probable that Violet is not shouting at the staff to be awkward but because the damage to her brain means that she believes she is once again that mother who needs to get her child ready for an appointment. From Violet's perspective the behaviour of the staff is ridiculous and incomprehensible. Imagine you had an important appointment and needed to get your child organised and someone came into the house and kept telling you to stop because it is dinner time. Under these circumstances would it be that unreasonable to get very annoyed with the person for preventing you from getting on? If they persisted in blocking you, would your frustration increase to the point that you may even think that physical intervention to get them out of the way was justified?

To understand people with dementia it is crucial to engage with their belief system rather than focus on bringing them back to 'agreed reality'. If you really believe something but no-one else will believe you, this is extremely distressing. It is normal to react to invalidation either with anger and aggression or with despair and hopelessness. People with dementia are no different to anyone else in this respect. They are only different in so far as brain damage makes 'agreed reality' unattainable. Once the hippocampus is damaged, trying to get people to re-learn lost information through reality orientation or similar techniques is futile because there is no hippocampus left to 'catch' the information (although more modern uses of this technique as a cueing method to provide a perceptual boost (Holden and Stokes, 2002) can be helpful because it increases the chances of stable patterns forming within the knowledge networks of the association cortex). It is more productive to accept that the person's reality is changing and make the effort to adapt to their reality. To help Violet it is essential to engage with the primary, motivating belief, that Mary must be found, and help her gain closure. Violet will only be able to think about coming to dinner once she is satisfied that Mary is alright. Reiteration of the fact that it is dinner time fails to acknowledge her belief and results only in distress and opposition. The work of Stokes (2000) demonstrates that most challenging behaviour is not motivated by a desire to be difficult but is rather an expression of unmet need. The challenge is not simply to manage the behaviour but to go to the root of the behaviour and identify the need so that it can be met.

Neurological Impairment and Dementia Care Nursing: What are the Lessons?

The key message in this chapter is that people's experience of dementia arises, in part, from neurological impairments. The chapter clearly shows that it is important for nurses to understand the extent to which neurological impairments give rise to cognitive impairments. It is important to recognise the full extent of a person's neurological impairment so that should that person's reality begin to shift backwards into the past, nurses, and other health and social care professionals, stop trying to bring that person back into an 'agreed reality' of the present. Until treatments to arrest or reverse the underlying disease processes are developed, people with dementia are simply not capable of re-entering 'agreed reality' and to try and get them to do so is unrealistic and, therefore, unkind.

Rather, nurses should try to enter their reality and try to identify the beliefs and habits that motivate them. This is not easy but reminiscence work (Bruce et al. 1999), Resolution Therapy (Stokes, 2000) and Validation Therapy (Feil, 1992) provide useful techniques and structures through which nurses can learn to understand the world as perceived and interpreted by the person with dementia. Fundamental alterations in consciousness and belief are as inevitable a consequence of hippocampal and cortical damage as paralysis is of spinal damage. The nature of the neurological impairment means that people with dementia cannot be 'lectured' or 'coaxed' out of their cognitive impairments or 'drilled' back into agreed reality. Jokes about the things that people with dementia do or say reflect far more badly on the person making the joke than the person with dementia. Ageist or 'dementia-ist' attitudes must be challenged by a greater understanding of the nature of cognitive impairment within society as a whole.

The nature of the neurological impairment in dementia is very challenging. As a society we value cognitive skills very highly and are thus very afraid of cognitive impairment. Professionals need to understand that most people will not be able to accept and adapt to the cognitive symptoms of dementia without help and support. Nurses can make a significant contribution to this situation by working alongside people with dementia, and their families, to help them accept what is lost and to make the most of what remains. But what is lost is very significant and it is unlikely that either the person or their family can accept this without passing through the normal phases of bereavement. Nurses can support this process by being sensitive to the grief whilst also trying to generate realistic expectations about the kinds of relationship the family can expect to maintain with the person as the dementia advances (for example, that even if language is lost they can still maintain a positive relationship simply by being present, smiling, holding hands and using this time to celebrate the person's past life and achievements).

Summary

Despite the magnitude of the challenges posed by dementia, it is critical to maintain a positive attitude. This review has shown that although dementia is associated with damage to the highest regions of the cortex, much of the brain does remain functional. The world of the person with dementia is well summarised by Stokes (2000; p. 73):

> This is the subjective life of the person with dementia: a person who remains an active agent; an individual who makes decisions and initiates actions, while residing in a reality that resonates 'not knowing'; a person who as a consequence may be sorely misunderstood.

What this quotation makes clear is that behind the cognitive confusion remains an active person with a subjective life just like anyone else. It is unfair to support people with dementia enough to keep them alive, but not enough to respect the reality of their continued being. Thus, our approach to the neurological impairment must be one of profiling in which we not only identify and accept areas of weakness, but also identify areas of preservation and strength so that we can work positively with people with dementia, helping them live successfully with their disability.

References

Bayles, K. A., Tomeda, C. K., Kasniak, A. W. and Trosset M. W. (1991). Alzheimer's disease effects on semantic memory: loss of structure or impaired processing? *Journal of Cognitive Neuroscience* 3, 166–182.

Braak, H. and Braak, E. (1991) Neuropathological staging of Alzheimer-related changes. *Acta Neuropathologica* (Berlin) 82, 239–250.

Bruce, E., Hodgson, S. and Schweitzer, P. (1999) Reminiscing with People with Dementia. Age Exchange, London.

Damasio, A. R. (1994). *Descartes' Error*. London: Papermac.

DeLeon, M. J., Potegal, M. and Gurland B. (1984) Wandering and parietal signs in senile dementia of Alzheimer type. *Neuropsychobiology* 11, 155–157.

Feil, N. (1993). *The Validation Breakthrough: Simple Techniques for Communicating with People with Alzheimer's-type Dementia*. Baltimore: Health Professions Press.

Goodale, M. A., Milner, A. D., Jakabson, L. S. and Carey, D. P. (1993). A neurological dissociation between perceiving objects and grasping them. *Nature* 349, 154–156.

Haxby, V., Durra, R., Grady, C. L., Culter, N. R. and Rapaport, S. I. (1985). Relations between neuropsychological and cerebral metabolic asymmetries in early Alzheimer's disease. *Journal of Cerebral Blood Flow and Metabolism* 5, 193–200.

Hodges, J. R., Salmon, D. P. and Butters, N. (1992). Semantic memory impairment in Alzheimer's disease: Failure of access or degraded knowledge. *Neuropsychologia* 30, 301–314.

Hodges, J. R., Salmon, D. P. and Butters, N. (1993). Recognition and naming of famous faces in Alzheimer's disease: A cognitive analysis. *Neuropsychologia* 31, 775–788.

Holden, U. and Stokes, G. (2002). Neuropsychological impairments and rehabilitation approaches. In G. Stokes and F. Goudie (eds), *The essential dementia care handbook*. Bicester: Speechmark, 92–101.

Lamdon-Ralph, M. A., Ellis, A. W. and Franklin, S. (1995). Semantic loss without surface dyslexia. *Neurocase* 1, 363–369.

Lewis, D. A., Campbell, M. J., Terry, R. D. and Morrison, J. H. (1987). Laminar and regional distributions of neurofibrillary tangles and neuritic plaques in Alzheimer's disease: A quantitative study of visual and auditory cortices. *The Journal of Neuroscience* 7, 1799–1808.

Luria, A. R. (1973). *The working brain*. London: Penguin.

Martin, A. (1987). Representation of semantic and spatial knowledge in Alzheimer's patients: Implications for models of preserved learning in amnesia. *Journal of Clinical and Experimental Neuropsychology* 9, 191–224.

Martin, A. and Fedio, P. (1983). Word production and comprehension in Alzheimer's disease: The breakdown of semantic knowledge. *Brain and Language* 19, 124–141.

Murdoch, B. E., Chenery, H. J., Wilks, V. and Boyle, R. S. (1987). Language disorders in dementia of the Alzheimer type. *Brain and Language* 31, 122–137.

Neary, D. and Snowden, J. S. (2003). Causes of dementia in younger people. In R. C. Baldwin and M. Murray, *Younger People with Dementia*. London: Martin Dunitz, pp. 7–41.

Pearson, R. C. A., Esiri, M. M., Hions, R. W., Wilcock, G. K. and Powell, T. P. S. (1985). Anatomical correlates of the distribution of the pathological changes in the neocortex in Alzheimer's disease. *Proceedings of the National Academy of Sciences (USA)* 82, 4531–4534.

Powell, J. (2000). *Care to Communicate: Helping the Older Person with Dementia*. London: Hawker Publications.

Stokes, G. (2000). *Challenging Behaviour in Dementia*. Bicester: Speechmark.

Stokes, G. (2002). Wandering: We walk, they wander. In G. Stokes and F. Goudie (eds), *The Essential Dementia Care Handbook*. Bicester: Speechmark, 152–166.

WHO (2003). *International Statistical Classification of Diseases and Related Health Problems. 10th Revision Version for 2003 ed*. WHO: Geneva.

Chapter 5

The family's experience of dementia

Trevor Adams

Learning Outcomes

After reading the chapter you will be able to

- critically discuss what is meant by 'informal care' and its developments within dementia care;
- critically examine the relationship between 'informal care' and dementia care nursing;
- identify various ways of understanding informal care within dementia care;
- critically review different approaches towards the informal care of people with dementia;
- discuss the implications of informal care by different groups of people.

Introduction

Various approaches that highlight the experience of people with dementia have been discussed in Chapter 3, and provide worthwhile insights for nurses working alongside people with dementia. While these approaches are valuable, we believe they are too narrow and fail to fully capture what is happening between different people and agencies within dementia care settings. When someone has dementia, it is not just the person with dementia who is affected; others will also find themselves caught up in the experience, most notably other members of the family, including those seen as 'informal carers'. This chapter, therefore, examines the wider experience of different family members who are giving direct or indirect informal care to a relative with dementia.

Informal Care

The term 'informal carer' is generally taken to mean people caring for others in private dwelling places outside formal payment arrangements and whose relationship with the person with dementia is underpinned by obligations structured by marriage or family ties. Informal carers may comprise any member of the family and may come from the same generation, for example, husbands and wives, brothers and sisters, or may be trans-generational, such as sons and daughters. While the term 'informal carer' is typically used in health and social care, talking about 'informal carers' limits people's understanding as it is often not just the primary informal carer who is affected by a relative with dementia but the whole family! We would therefore prefer to think of various family members being affected by their relative with dementia, rather than just one specific family member acting as *the* informal carer.

The 'care for the carer' approach has flourished since the early 1980s and was supported by 'neo-liberal' social ideas that were implemented within social policy in the UK by the first Thatcher administration. One early area in which these ideas were implemented was with respect to community care, and gave rise to a shift from 'care *in* the community' to 'care *by* the community'. In this approach, informal carers are seen as an indigenous form of support in communities. This position was initially put into place in the government document *Growing Older* (DHSS, 1981), which stated:

> [T]he primary sources of support and care for elderly people are informal and voluntary. These spring from the personal ties of kinship, friendship and neighbourhood. ... It is the role of public authorities to sustain and where necessary, develop – never to replace – such support and care. (p. 3)

The full effect of these ideas may be seen in *The Carers (Services and Recognition) Act, 1995*, (DH 1995) which gave all informal carers the right to have a separate and independent assessment of their needs, and *The Carers National Strategy* (DH, 1999).

This approach continues to underpin policy documents like *Everybody's Business* (DH, 2005), which affirms the informal care given by family members and recognises that the many informal carers are old themselves so that, while care may be rewarding, it is often emotionally and physically demanding and may cause financial hardship. *Everybody's Business* notes that 'Carers can be isolated, and less able to take part in the employment and social activities that they previously employed' (DH, 2005, p. 5).

The 'Rise' of Informal Care

When I first worked in dementia care nursing in the late 1970s, not many people talked about informal carers. This did not mean that they did not exist. Studies by Sheldon (1948) and Townsend (1963) clearly reveal that families at that time often looked after their older, dependent relatives. However, the care that was given was hidden and private, and never highlighted. Typically, informal care was subsumed into family life or taken for granted as part of the work of women within the family. Over the past 25 years, however, the contribution of informal care within social policy has increasingly been recognised within society and government policy, and is now an important cornerstone of health and social care provision.

Informal 'carers' or 'caregivers' as they are called in North America comprise family members, friends and neighbours. It is now commonplace to think a person can only have one informal carer. However, this is frequently not the case and often there is more than one relative providing 'hands-on' care, while other family members are providing indirect support. Keith (1995) in a study of informal care to people with dementia found that it was quite common for more than one family member to provide informal care, and that responsibility was often shared between different family members. Often informal care is provided by female members of the family such as wives, daughters and daughters-in-law. However, often husbands and sons are also involved in providing informal care, and their contribution and special needs should be acknowledged (Arber and Gilbert, 1989).

Various criticisms of informal care have emerged (Bytheway and Johnson, 1998; Lloyd, 2000; Parker and Clarke, 2002; Stalker, 2003). First, informal care has been seen as merely a way of reducing government expenditure. Second, it has been argued that informal care is based on a traditional understanding of the role of women in the family. This role is now out of date, as many have responsibilities outside the home. Thus informal care is summed up by the equation: informal care = family care = female care (Land, 1978) and leads to women frequently experiencing too much physical and emotional stress. Third, various conceptual and methodological difficulties have been identified in informal care such as it was driven by anecdotal accounts, a lack of theorising about carers, an assumption that carers and users have shared interests and needs, a neglect of the different types of carers, a focus upon the 'burden' of care and the restrictions upon the carer's life, a failure to acknowledge pockets of 'hidden carers', and the absence of 'users accounts' (Stalker, 2003).

Informal Caregiving to People with Dementia

As we have already discussed, the 'rise of the carer' led to a burgeoning amount of knowledge about the provision of informal care to a range of people, including people with dementia. A number of approaches were developed that explain the nature of informal care to people with dementia (see George, 2005).

One of these approaches was concerned with the idea of stress. Early models of stress highlighted a direct relationship between people's experience of stress and stress-provoking behaviours. The idea here is that a particular behaviour, such as incontinence or wandering, would elicit a degree of stress in the informal carer. This model was developed by Cannon (1932) and was called 'the engineering model of stress' because, as in the physical sciences, people's experience of stress was directly related to the strain they encountered.

Transactional Approaches to Stress within Informal Care

This 'engineering model' was eventually abandoned in favour of a transactional approach towards stress in which people's subjective experience of stress is mediated by various psychological and social phenomena (Nolan and Grant, 1992). DeLongis and O'Brien (1990) adopt this approach towards informal carers to people with dementia by drawing on the work of Lazarus and Folkman (1984), who argue that people's adaptation to stress is mediated by their appraisal of the stressor and also their coping strategies. They outline two forms of appraisal. First, primary appraisal, which is concerned with what is at stake for the person in terms of harm/loss, threat or challenge. Second, secondary appraisal, which considers what can be done to manage the problem. In addition, Lazarus and Folkman (1984) identify two styles of coping: 'emotion-focused' strategies which are primarily cognitive processes concerned with lessening emotional distress, and 'problem-focused' strategies associated with solving problems through processes such as problem identification, generating alternative solutions, weighing up the evidence, making a choice and acting.

Stressful Events

A number of important studies were published in the 1980s that revealed the stress experienced by family carers to people with dementia. Sanford (1975), for example, identified the main problems they experience, which included nocturnal wandering, faecal incontinence, an inability to wash, dress or feed unaided, immobility and risky behaviour such as using a gas cooker.

Donaldson et al. (1997), in a review of studies published between 1980 and 1995, found evidence to support a link between certain symptoms of dementia and their negative impact upon carers. Non-cognitive symptoms of dementia, including hallucinations, sadness and aggression, were more likely to contribute to the carers' experience of burden.

Morris et al. (1988) concluded that there is broad agreement between studies concerning what behavioural alterations are more likely to be reported as problems and comprise incontinence, over-demanding behaviour and the need for constant supervision. Moreover, the psychological health of carers depended upon a combination of the degree of dependency or difficulty of the older person; the state of the carer's own health; and the closeness of the present or past relationship between themselves and the person with dementia.

The Psychological and Physical Well-being of Carers to People with Dementia

Various studies used the General Health Questionnaire [GHQ] (Goldberg, 1978) to measure the impact of informal care upon the psychological well-being of carers. These studies have consistently shown an association between carers' scores on the GHQ and specific problems experienced by carers. For example, Levin et al. (1989) found that the higher the number of major problems experienced by carers – incontinence, night disturbance, unsafe acts, lack of purposeful activity, trying behaviours and the inability to hold a normal conversation – the higher the carer's GHQ scores.

Mediating Factors
'Social' mediators of stress

Other studies have also identified various 'social' factors that affect carers' experience of stress. Ballard et al. (1995) found that carers

who were depressed and were living with the person who had
dementia were particularly vulnerable to the experience of stress.
Studies vary in the amount of stress that these social phenomena
contribute. Indeed, Gilhooly (1984, 1986) found that the only characteristic of the person with dementia that was significantly associated with the carer's morale was gender, and found that carers of
women with dementia had better morale and mental health than
those caring for men who had dementia. It has also been found that
male carers were more likely to have higher morale than female
carers (Gilhooly, 1984).

Family Relationships and Structure

A number of studies have examined the relationship between the
amount of stress that informal carers encounter and various characteristics of the family. Boss (2002) found that certain features of a
family, particularly who is included inside and outside the family
boundary, have a significant effect on carers' experience of stress.
She argues that when a family member develops dementia they are
bodily present in the family but psychologically absent, and this
leads to family members experiencing stress that arises from
'ambiguous loss'.

A number of studies within dementia care have drawn on the
work of Vaughn and Leff (1976) on expressed emotion in families
containing people with schizophrenia. They understand 'expressed
emotion' as behaviours that display the emotional status of family
members. Bledin et al. (1990) found that expressed emotion was displayed by carers who experienced a greater level of emotional stress.

Gilhooly and Whittock (1998) found that carer stress was positively associated with a number of characteristics, such as the
carer's gender, psychological well-being, amount of contact with
friends and the quality of the relationship between the carer and the
person with dementia. This latter finding corresponds with various
studies that highlight the contribution that other family characteristics make to carers' experience of stress, such as closeness and affection (Horowitz and Shindelman, 1983), mutuality (Hirschfield,
1981) and marital intimacy (Morris et al., 1988). These studies suggest that 'the family' is a more appropriate frame of reference than
simply informal carers since one person in the family having
dementia means all the members of the family are likely to be
affected.

Coping

Pearlin et al. (1990) identify three types of coping strategy used by carers to people with dementia: (1) minimising the burden upon the carer; (2) managing the meaning of the situation; (3) managing symptoms of distress that arise in the caregivers. Pruncho and Resch (1989) examine various coping strategies to people with dementia and the effect they have upon the emotional well-being of carers to people with dementia. They found that carers who used coping strategies relating to 'acceptance', such as 'making the best of it', had lower levels of depression.

In addition, Pruncho and Resch (1989) found that carers using instrumental coping strategies such as 'doing something new to solve the situation' and 'making a plan of action' had higher levels of positive affect with no association of depression. However, they found that carers who used coping strategies such as 'wishfulness,' for example, carers who wished that they could change the way they 'felt', and 'interpsychic' coping strategies, such as carers who resorted to day dreaming and imagining a better time and place than their present situation, had lower levels of positive affect.

Appraisal

A number of studies of carers for people with dementia have found that the attributional style of carers affects their experience of stress. Pagel et al. (1985) found that carers who perceived a loss of control in their situation were consistently found to have higher levels of depression. Morris et al. (1988) found that the carer's perceived loss of control is frequently a negative feature of caregiving. Morris et al. (1989) found a very high correlation between both (1) an increased sense of control in the carer relating to their perceived control over their spouse's behaviour, and (2) their own emotional reactions and low levels of depression and sense of strain. Carers' perceptions of the patients' everyday functioning and dysphoria directly influenced their perception of caregiving as a burden.

The significance of carers' appraisals and interpretations of their situation has been supported in recent studies. Levesque et al. (1995) asked carers about the severity and behaviour of the people with dementia for whom they were caring and the degree to which they found these features disturbing. They found that with particular impairments and behaviours, such as difficulties with activities of living, the person with dementia becoming depressed or having behavioural or memory problems, it was the carers' feelings, rather than the level of severity in the person with dementia that was related to poor psychological well-being on the carers' part.

There are various problems with 'stress and coping' approaches towards informal care. The first problem is that they imply that caring for a relative with dementia is always stressful, never rewarding and satisfying. Motenko (1989) in a study of 50 older women caring for husbands with dementia at home found that some women found caregiving gratifying, and it was associated with continuing activities that husbands and wives had previously undertaken and maintaining meaningful relationships.

The second problem is that they tend to pathologise the carer and construct caregiving as having a detrimental effect on the carer's health and well-being.

Third, the approach provides few insights into the feelings of the person with dementia. Usually, 'stress and coping' approaches models tend to construct people with dementia as having a disease and being a burden to their carer.

Loss and Grief Models of Informal Caregiving

Carers sometimes talk about giving care to people with dementia as a 'living bereavement' (Taylor, 1987) and say that their relative is no longer the person they once knew; they have lost them to dementia. The idea that carers experience a sense of loss has been acknowledged by researchers and professionals for some time (see Barnes et al., 1981). Various studies have identified different aspects of the carer's experience of loss and grief (Loos and Bowd 1997; Moyle et al. 2002).

Jones and Martinson (1992) found that carers expressed four different types of pre-death experience: intense during caregiving; death as a relief; readiness to go and readiness to get on with life. Using a larger sample, Collins et al. (1993) examined the experience of loss and grief experienced by family carers before and following the death of their relative with dementia. The sample comprised 350 people providing informal care to a relative with dementia. Of these, 82 of the relatives died during the study and thus additional data was available about the carer's post-death experience. The study identified six themes.

Loss of Familiarity and Intimacy

A predominant theme expressed by carers was that the dementia had taken away the person they had once known.

Over 33% said that there had been a fundamental change in their relationship with the person who now had dementia. Carers expressed the belief that difficulties in communication are one way that caring for someone with dementia is different from caring for someone with another long-term mental health problem.

Loss of Hope

Nearly half of the carers in the study said that they were aware that there was going to be an inevitable decline in their relationship owing to dementia. Carers continued to remain intensely involved in caring for their relative even after they had lost hope that there would be a recovery.

'You are watching and watching, wondering what will happen next to take more of the person you love away'.

Awareness that there was going to be no recovery was often accompanied by expressions of helplessness and talk about how long the dementia has lasted.

Pre-death Grief

Nearly half of the carers in the study said that they had felt grief before their relative had died, 'I did all my grieving before my wife died. Every day I lost a little piece of her.' The study found that carers used particularly vivid ways of talking about their experience of caregiving that touched every aspect of their existence.

Expectancy of Death

Over 25% of the carers in the study talked about how they had expected death, though feelings of shock were expressed when death actually came.

Comments about the peacefulness and calmness of the death were common in the carers whose relative had died.

Post-death Grief

Most of the carers in the study who had experienced their relative's death had experienced a sense of emotional relief. This relief was often on behalf of the person with dementia. Feelings of relief often were accompanied by feelings of loneliness and grief.

Caregiving reflections
After the death of their spouse many of the carers expressed doubts about the decisions they had made about their relative's care. Regret was experienced by nearly a quarter of the carers whose relative had died, even though they acknowledged how much care they have already provided. Many carers, however, identified the importance of their role and the meaning they found in it.

Models of Informal Care and Service Provision

Various studies have discussed the relationship between informal carers and the people for whom they care. Twigg and Atkin (1995) have put forward an influential model that identified four patterns of professional engagement with informal carers.

- *Carers as resources* – the predominant model which employs a wide understanding of who is a carer and sees them in general as free, available, preferred sources of family support. They exist separately from statutory provision, which may have to step in when such care is not or is no longer available.
- *Carers as co-workers* – working with or alongside professionals, carers carry out tasks and their work interweaves with formal systems of support. Carers' needs are met and they are able to continue with the job.
- *Carers as co-clients* – being supported in their own right by services which attempt to provide relief. The carers' needs and well-being are a key focus of support. The problems of the carer are considered and responded to, even if this may divert attention away from the person being cared for.
- *Superseded carers* – the aim is not to support the caregiving but to transcend or supersede it. Often referred to as 'relatives' or 'family members', they are seen as distinct from the person to whom carer is being given; indeed there may be a conflict of interest between the two. Services may help support such carers and the person to whom care is being given by starting the healthy process of separation.

Twigg and Atkin (1995, p. 10) identify various models relating to the negotiation of services and highlight three different attitudes that informal carers may have towards their role. The first attitude relates to families that are engulfed and are so over-whelmed by what is happening that help is perceived as unsuit-able or threatening. In the second attitude, carers can consider their position and the boundaries they may wish to choose, and begin to plan. The third attitude relates to symbiosis and sees carers as identifying themselves with the person who has the dis-ability or illness and are unwilling to relinquish responsibility. Unlike carers who set boundaries and are open to assistance, and may indeed make demands on systems and professionals, those in a symbolic symbiotic state are presented as generally content with services unless they de-stabilise their way of doing things or the relationship.

The work of Twigg and Atkin (1994) is helpful here as it outlines various possible configurations between carers and professionals. Manthorpe et al. (2003) argue that the way Twigg and Atkin (1994) understand caregiving is problematic because professionals' responses to carers are not simply a matter of transactions, but rather are mediated by assumptions on both sides. However, what should be noted is that Twigg and Atkin (1994) make little mention of the extent to which the people who are receiving informal care, in our case people with dementia, are participating in the negotiation of services.

Temporal Approaches to Caregiving

Various studies provide evidence about the changing circumstances and subjective experience of informal carers to people with dementia (Wilson, 1989; Willoughby and Keating, 1991). Some stud-ies, however, examine more specific aspects of caregiving such as the impact on wives who receive the diagnosis that their husband has dementia (Morgan and Laing, 1991) and social processes associ-ated with people making decisions about relatives with dementia (Wakerbath, 1999).

A more sophisticated model has been developed by Keady (1999), who charts out the typical progression taken by informal carers to people with dementia. Initially, Keady draws on the work of Eraut (1994) and argues that as they provide care carers learn new skills by a process of trial and error, and through continued caregiving they develop expertise. Then Keady develops the main part of his thesis, which comprises an outline of different transitions carers make as they provide informal care to the person with dementia.

Building on the Past
Keady points out that strictly speaking 'building on the past' is not a stage. He supports its inclusion as a legitimate stage within the caregiving process because of its importance before, during and after the provision of informal care. Keady argues that to understand the interpersonal dynamics between the person with dementia and their informal carer it is important to understand their past relationship.

Recognising the Need
This stage occurs when carers become aware of the changing relationship between themselves and the person with dementia. Included within this stage are a number of sub-stages. The first comprises 'noticing' when some of the cared-for person's behaviour catches the carer's attention. Keady argues that initially carers want to normalise these aberrant behaviours and search for logical explanations about what has happened. Eventually, depending on how aberrant the behaviour actually is, the carer will begin to suspect that something is amiss and the carer changes from thinking that 'things are OK' to 'this might be serious'. This situation might lead the carer to find out what other family members think or might even check it out with the person who has dementia themselves! During this period, the carers may find themselves keeping an ever-vigilant eye on their relative with dementia.

This stage leads on to the next in which carers seek 'confirmation' from other people that something really is wrong. Usually carers seek the advice of the General Practitioner [GP]. Keady says that frequently GPs are often offhand with carers and are sometimes dismissive. When this occurs, the carers will find themselves returning to the situation from which they started. When this happens carers are likely to feel that they are 'banging their head against a brick wall' and this will inhibit further contact with professional agencies. It is only when further crises occur that the carer will find themselves in a position that they are able to go to a health care worker again. At this time a 'diagnostic quest' (Corbin and Strauss, 1988) is occurring and may lead to a period of 'diagnostic limbo' between suspicion and confirmation about the diagnosis. This period is highly ambiguous and, as a result, is very stressful. It is not until certainty appears through a diagnosis that this stage can end and the carer can proceed to the next stage of 'taking it on'.

Taking It on

This stage begins when there is a cognitive shift within the carer towards more formally recognising their role as that of a carer. Even though it is a crucial stage that all family members who become carers need to pass, sometimes they fall into it as part of a continuation of existing relationships. Sometimes tensions may arise between nurses and carers, for example, when a carer refuses to let their relative take up a place at a Day Hospital or when the nurse does not share the carer's concerns.

Working through It

This stage denotes the carers' active work to provide care and is developed from the metaphor of 'work' developed by Corbin and Strauss (1988). In this stage carers become experts, particularly in the day-to-day aspects of caregiving as they maximise the positive elements while minimising the negative.

Reaching the End

This stage occurs when the instrumental part of caregiving has ceased; in no way does it imply that the carer ceases to care. The stage may occur in a number of ways and would include a person with dementia entering a residential care home. Keady points out that entry into this stage is often sudden and the carer has little professional support to deal with the painful emotions that may arise at this time, such as guilt and anxiety.

A New Beginning

This occurs when carers cease undertaking instrumental care and have a new life. The carer must not forget the past, but build on it to create a new beginning. This stage is successfully accomplished by the family creating a balanced perception of what they have achieved during caring, recognising the value of their effort over the years and coming to a realisation that the choice of alternative residential care is the most appropriate.

Informal Care within Gay, Lesbian, Bisexual and Transsexual Couples

Most studies on informal care have not differentiated between straight and gay carers. However, there is now an increasing recognition of the differences in the provision of informal care between various non-dominant groups in society such as people who come from ethnically different groups and those who are gay, lesbian or transsexual. Ward (2000) argues that social policy has assumed that people are within traditional families. This has led many people who are gay or lesbian not revealing their sexuality, as they are afraid that it might lead to discrimination and stigmatisation. Ward (2000) describes the difficulties partners may have with services who find it difficult to accept their position as the partner of the person with dementia and thus not take their role as a family carer seriously. The Alzheimer's Society in the UK has developed a web site for Lesbian, Gay, Bisexual and Transgender (LGBT) carers and offers is a telephone support service for anyone who is lesbian, gay, bisexual or transgender and who is, or who has been, caring for someone with dementia. They also, publish a newsletter which is of interest to people with dementia, and their partners (See gay-http://www.alzheimers.org.uk/Gay_Carers/index.htm) [accessed 5th July 2007].

Informal Care and Ethnicity

Everybody's Business (DH, 2005) highlights the increasing need for services to be culturally appropriate to older people and their carers. A number of studies have highlighted the experience of carers to people with dementia from black and minority ethnic groups (Adamson, 2001). Turner et al. (2005) found that South Asian older people had much less specific knowledge about dementia and were much more likely to see dementia as part of the normal ageing process. They were less likely to think that there were treatments available and were more likely to think that care should be provided by family or friends. These studies reveal that the experiences of people with dementia and their family members show that the important issues for nurses include language, religious belief and observance, cultural practices (including food and personal care practices) and social support and coping mechanisms. Illiffe and Manthorpe (2004) argue that all health and social care providers, including nurses, should recognise the diversity of people with dementia and increase access to appropriate quality mainstream person-centred services, rather than develop segregated or specialised services.

Informal Care in Rural Areas

People with dementia and their family carers living in rural areas may encounter particular difficulties because of their social isolation and remoteness (Innes, 2003). Buettner and Langrish (1999) in a study of family carers found that rural carers were often older than carers in urban areas and that they used fewer services. Integration into community networks has been found to be an advantage and a positive relationship has been found between older people's perceived health status, with their social network and level of social support. The stigma associated with having dementia may further diminish a sense of belonging to social networks for people living in rural areas. Resistance to help and withdrawing from public activities may contribute to carer's feelings of remoteness, and the closeness of rural communities may be a barrier to diagnosis.

Summary

This chapter has focused on the experience of family members who offer informal carer to people with dementia. The chapter has critically reviewed different approaches towards the provision of informal care by family members. While there are many similarities between the experiences of different family carers, there are some special circumstances that make each carer's experience different. The key role played by informal carers within decision-making is emphasised by *Everybody's Business* (DH, 2005).

Highlighting the needs of family carers raises important questions about the position of family carers with respect to the person with dementia. There is a possibility that by bringing the carer into focus, the person with dementia will become vague and fuzzy and their wishes and choices ignored. Focusing on the carer allows their relative with dementia to seem passive and that they are unable contribute to decisions about their own care. We would challenge approaches that highlight the person with dementia at the expense of the person with dementia and would argue that the carer's experience cannot be understood in isolation from that of the person with dementia and that there should be an equal recognition of the person with dementia and their informal carer(s) in dementia care nursing.

References

Adamson, J. (2003). Awareness and understanding of dementia in African/Caribbean and South Asian families. *Health and Social Care in the Community* 9, 6, 391–396.

Arber, S. and Gilbert, N. (1989). Men: the forgotten carers. *Sociology* 23, 1, 111–118.

Ballard, C. G., Saad, K., Coope, B., Graham, C., Gahir, M., Wilcock, G. K. and Oyebode, F. (1995). The aetiology of depression in the carers of dementia sufferers. *Journal of Affective Disorders* 35, 1, 59–63.

Barnes, R., Raskind, M., Scott, M. and Murphy, C. (1981). Problems of families caring for Alzheimer patients: use of a support group. *Journal of the American Geriatrics Society* 29, 80–85.

Bledin, K. D., MacCarthy, B., Kuipers, L. and Woods R. T. (1990). Daughters of people with dementia: expressed emotion, strain and coping. *British Journal of Psychiatry* 157, 221–227.

Boss, P. (2002). *Family Stress Management: A Contextual Approach.* (2nd ed.) London: Sage.

Bowes, A. and Wilkinson, H. (2003). We didn't know it would get that bad': South Asian experiences of dementia and the service response. *Health and Social Care in the Community* 11, 5, pp. 387–396.

Buettner, L. L. and Langrish, S. (1999). Rural vs. urban caregivers of older adults with probable Alzheimer's Disease: Perceptions regarding daily living and recreation needs. In M. J. Keller (ed.) *Caregiving – Leisure and Aging,* New York: Haworth Press, Inc., pp. 51–65.

Bytheway, B. and Johnson, J. (1998). The social construction of 'carers'. In A. Symonds and A. Kelly (eds) *The Social Construction of Community Care.* Basingstoke: Macmillan.

Cannon, W. B. (1932). *The Wisdom of the Body.* New York: Norton.

Collins, C., Liken, M., King, S. and Kokinakis, C. (1993). Loss and grief among family caregivers of relatives with dementia. *Qualitative Health Research* 3, 2, 236–253.

Corbin, J. M. and Strauss, A. (1988). *Unending Work and care: Mapping Chronic Illness at Home.* San Francisco, CA: Jossey Bass.

DeLongis, A. and O'Brien, T. (1990). An interpersonal framework for stress and coping: an application to families of Alzheimer's disease. In M. Stephens, J. Crowther, S. Hobfoll and I. Tennenbaum. (eds) *Stress and Coping in Later-Life Families.* New York: Hemisphere.

Department of Health (1981) *Growing Older.* London: HMSO.

Department of Health (1995). *Carers (Recognition and Services) Act.* London: HMSO.

Department of Health (1999). *The Carers National Strategy.* London: HMSO.

Department of Health (2005). *Everybody's Business. Integrated Mental Health Services for Older Adults: A Service Development Guide.* London: Care Services Improvement Partnership (CSIP).

Donaldson, C., Tarrier, N. and Burns, A. (1997). The impact of the symptoms of dementia on caregivers. *British Journal of Psychiatry* 170, 62–68.

Eraut, M. (1994). *Developing Professional Knowledge and Competence.* London: Falmer.

George, L. K. (2005). Stress and Coping. In M. L. Johnson (ed.) *The Cambridge Handbook of Age and Ageing.* Cambridge: Cambridge University Press. pp. 292–300.

Gilhooly, M. L. M. (1984). The impact of caregiving on caregivers: factors associated with the psychological well-being of people supporting a dementing relative in the community. *British Journal of Medical Psychology* 59, 165–171.

Gilhooly, M. L. M. (1986). Emotional stress among supporters of the elderly mentally infirm. *British Journal of Psychiatry* 145, 172–177.

Gilhooly, M. L. M. and Whittick, J. E. (1998). Expressed emotion in caregivers of the dementing elderly. *British Journal of Medical Psychology* 62, 3, 265–272.

Gilleard, C. J., Belford, H., Gilleard, E., Whittick, J. E. and Gledhill, K. (1984). Emotional stress amongst the supporters of the elderly mentally infirm. *British Journal of Psychiatry* 145, 172–177.

Goldberg, D. (1978). *A manual for the General Health Questionnaire.* Windsor: NEFR Nelson.

Hirschfield, M. J. (1981). Families living and coping with the cognitively impaired. In A. Copp (ed.) *Recent Advances in Nursing, Volume. 2: Care of the Aged.* Edinburgh: Churchill Livingstone.

Horowitz, A and Shindelman, L. W. (1983). Reciprocity and affection: past influences to current caregiving. *Journal of Gerontological Social Work* 5, 5–20

Iliffe, S. and Manthorpe, J. (2004). The debate on ethnicity and dementia: from category fallacy to person-centred care? *Aging and Mental Health* 8, 4, 283–292.

Innes, A., Blackstock, K. Mason, A. Smith, A. and Cox, S. (2005). Dementia care provision in rural Scotland: service users' and carers' experiences. *Health and Social Care in the Community*, 13, 4, 354–365.

Jones, P. and Martinson, I. (1992) The experience of bereavement in caregivers of family members with Alzheimer's disease. *Image* 24, 172–176

Keady, J. (1999). *The Dynamics of Dementia: A Modified Grounded Theory Study.* PhD Thesis. Bangor: University of Wales.

Keith, C. (1995). Family caregiving systems: models, resources and values. *Journal of Marriage and the Family* 57, 179–189.

Land, H. (1978). Who cares for the family? *Journal of Social Policy* 7, 275–284.

Lazarus, R. S. and Folkman, S. (1984). *Stress, Appraisal and Coping*. New York: Springer.

Lloyd, L. (2000). Caring about carers: only half the picture? *Critical Social Policy* 20, 136–150.

Levesque, L., Cossette, S. and Laurin, L. (1995). A multi-dimensional examination of the psychological and social well-being of caregivers of a demented relative. *Research on Aging* 17, 3, 332–360.

Levin, E., Sinclair, I. and Gorbach, P. (1989). *Families, Services and Confusion in Old Age*. Alders hot: Avebury.

Loos, C. and Bowd, A. (1997). Caregivers to persons with Alzheimer's disease: some neglected implications of the experience of personal grief. *Death Studies* 21, 501–514.

Manthorpe, J., Ilife, S. and Eden, A. (2003). Testing Twigg and Atkin's typology of caring: a study of primary care professionals' perceptions of dementia care using a modified focus group method. *Health and Social Care in the Community* 11, 6, 477–485.

Morgan, D. G. and Laing, G. (1991). The diagnosis of Alzheimer's disease: the spouses experiences. *Qualitative Health Research* 1, 3, 370–387.

Morris, R. G., Morris, L. W. and Britton, P. G. (1988). Factors affecting the emotional well-being of the caregivers of dementia sufferers. *British Journal of Psychiatry* 153, 147–156.

Morris, R. G. Morris, L. W. and Britton, P. G. (1988). Factors affecting the emotional wellbeing of caregivers of dementia sufferers. *British Journal of Psychiatry* 153, 147–156.

Motenko, A. K. (1989). The frustrations, gratifications and well-being of dementia caregivers. *Gerontologist* 29, 2, 166–172.

Moyle, W., Edwards, H. and Clinton, M. (2002). Living with loss: Dementia and the family caregiver. *Australian Journal of Advanced Nursing* 19, 3, 25–31.

Nolan. M. and Grant, G. (1992). *Regular Respite*. London: Age Concern England.

Pagel, M. D. Becker, J. and Coppel, D. B. (1985). Loss of self-control, self-blame and depression: an investigation of spouse caregivers of Alzheimer's disease patients. *Journal of Abnormal Psychology* 94, 169–156.

Parker, G. and Clarke, H. (2002). Making the ends meet: do carers and disabled people have a common agenda? *Policy and Politics* 30, 3, 347–358.

Pearlin, L. I., Turner, H. and Semple, S. (1990). Coping and the mediation of stress. In Light, E., Lebowitz, B. D. (eds) *Alzheimer's Disease, Treatment and Stress: Directions for Research*. New York: Hemisphere Publishing. pp. 198–217.

Pruncho, R. A. and Resch, N. L. (1989). Aberrant behaviours and Alzheimer's disease: Mental health effects on spouse caregivers. *Journal of Gerontology* 39, 230–239.

Sanford, J. R. A. (1975). Tolerance of disability in elderly dependents by supporters at home: its significance for hospital practice. *British Medical Journal* iii, 471–475.

Sheldon, J. H. (1948). *The Social Medicine of Old Age: Report of an Inquiry in Wolverhampton*. Oxford: Oxford University Press.

Stalker, K. (2003). *Reconceptualising Work with 'Carers': New Directions for Policy and Practice*. London: Jessica Kingsley Publishers.

Taylor, P. (1987). A living bereavement. *Nursing Times* 83, 30, 27–30.

Townsend, P. (1963). *The Family Life of Old People*. Harmondsworth: Pelican.

Twigg, J. and Atkin, K. (1994). *Carers Perceived: Policy and Practice*. Buckingham: Open University Press.

Turner, S., Christie, A. and Haworth, E. (2005). South Asian and white older people and dementia: a qualitative study of knowledge and attitudes. *Diversity in Health and Social Care* 2, 3, 197–209.

Vaughn, C. and Leff, J. (1976). The measurement of expressed emotion in the families of psychiatric patients. *British Journal of Clinical Psychology* 15, 157–165.

Wackerbath, S. (1999). Modelling a dynamic decision process: supporting the decisions of caregivers of family members with dementia. *Qualitative Health Research* 9, 3, 294–314.

Ward, R. (2000). Waiting to be heard – dementia and the gay community. *Journal of Dementia Care* May/June, 24–25.

Wilson, H. S. (1989). Family caregiving for a relative with Alzheimer's dementia: coping with negative choices. *Nursing Research* 38, 2, 94–98.

Willoughby, J. and Keating, N. (1991). Being in control: the process of caring for a relative with Alzheimer's disease. *Qualitative Health Research* 1, 1, 27–50.

Chapter 6

Nursing people with dementia and their family members – towards a whole systems approach

Trevor Adams

Learning Outcomes

After reading the chapter you will be able to

- identify the key people involved with people who have dementia;
- describe various types of 'dyadic' interaction between the person with dementia and their primary informal carer;
- critically review the contribution of 'triadic' approaches towards dementia care nursing particularly, with 'relationship-centred care';
- outline various systems that may contribute towards the experience of people with dementia;
- evaluate the contribution of a whole systems approach towards dementia care nursing.

Introduction

In previous chapters we have seen how recent approaches towards the person with dementia and their informal carers have marginalised either the informal carer or the person with dementia. This situation is problematic not only because it leads to a fragmented approach towards dementia care but also because it fails to offer a understanding of how people with dementia and their family members work together. This situation has recently been resolved by the development of a broader basis for practice within documents that include *From Values to Action* (DH, 2006) and *Rights, Relationships and Recovery* (Scottish Executive, 2006). These documents move beyond an individualisation of dementia care as occurs in person-centred care or approaches that focus on the informal carer and brings into view the person with dementia *and* their carer. We would support this approach and this chapter examines various dyadic, triadic and systemic approaches that may be used to underpin dementia care nursing.

Dyadic Approaches towards Dementia Care

Dyadic approaches towards dementia care nursing highlight the relationship between two people. Within dementia care nursing dyadic approaches often characterise care that is offered in hospitals and residential nursing homes in which the focus is on the person with dementia and the nurse. However, as the provision of dementia care has increasingly moved from 'the hospital' to 'the community', interest has developed in the relationship between the person with dementia and their primary informal carer. This latter approach towards dementia care nursing is displayed in the work of Keady (1999), Helleström (2005) and Robinson et al. (2005).

Keady and the Idea of 'Working' by Couples in Which One Person Has Dementia

Keady (1999) offers a useful study of dyadic relationships within families containing people with dementia, and describes four main types of 'working' that occur between couples where one has dementia.

Working Together

Working together describes the optimal situation in which the person with dementia and their carer have a shared and early recognition of the clinical features of dementia. Help is jointly sought and received and the couples begin to make the best of the situation, together. In working together, there is a considerable amount of discussion and agreement between couples about the best possible way to move forward.

Working Alone

Working alone occurs when the person with dementia or their spouse work in isolation. This pattern usually occurs soon after the onset of dementia when the person with dementia is 'trying to cover their tracks' by hiding their symptoms. However, it may also occur in the latter stages of dementia when the carer can no longer engage with the person who has dementia. When working alone, carers and people with dementia often feel as though they are not receiving enough professional help.

Working Separately

This occurs when the person with dementia and their carer are engaged in separate and different processes: one covering their tracks and the other suspecting that there is something wrong and becoming increasingly vigilant trying to confirm these suspicions. Each party invests considerable effort into 'working separately' which may give rise to an emotionally fraught time with underlying tensions.

Working Apart

Working apart occurs when there has been a longstanding poor relationship between the person with dementia and their carer or when difficulties with 'working separately' have led to strained interactions. The person with dementia and their partner cannot reach a mutually agreed plan about how they can move the situation forward, and so they 'work apart'. Their relationship deteriorates and the carer increasingly feels as though they are trapped in their role. 'Working apart' captures the nature of relationships when managing the early adjustment process as attempts are made by both parties to understand the changing reality. This situation may be resolved in various ways, such as through open confirmation or a 'confrontative confirmation' in which the carer challenges the person with dementia.

Helleström and the Idea of 'Couplehood'

Keady's work has been developed by Helleström et al., (2005a, b) whose study comprised 132 interviews with 20 different couples. Each partner was interviewed separately, though a few were interviewed together. While Helleström et al. (2005a, b) warn against generalising from the sample, it is nevertheless possible for practitioners to gain insights. The key idea in the work of Helleström et al. (2005a, b) is 'couplehood'.

The first part of the study comprised an analysis of the first two sets of interviews (n = 74). The analysis revealed themes that were contained in the data which were found to be consistent with theoretical perspectives of the 'dynamics of dementia' (Keady, 1999) and work undertaken on 'awareness theory' by Hutchinson et al. (1997). This latter paper suggests that open awareness was preferable in families containing people with dementia and results in less discord between family members and offers more opportunities for psychological and spiritual closure. However, Hellström et al. (2005a, 2005b) found that rather than adopting an 'open awareness context', the couples actively fostered a more uncertain understanding in which there was 'mutual acknowledgement' that dementia existed but that the main focus of the spouses' effort was on making life as meaningful as possible. The data revealed that the husbands and wives in the study worked together as a couple rather than as individuals and that they attempted to create and sustain what she termed as a 'nurturative relational context' in which the two main goals are to (1) sustain the quality of the spouses' relationship and (2) maintain the self-image and sense of agency of the person with dementia.

The second part of the study examined the nature of the 'nurturative relational context'. Following further analysis of the data it was found that one of the couple's primary goal was to 'do things together' for as long as possible as a means of maintaining the quality of life of each partner. This desire was based on a mutual appreciation of the continuing value of their relationship. The analysis revealed that over time the partner without the dementia had to take on increasing responsibility as their partner's ability to 'maintain involvement' reduced. The analysis showed that 'doing things together', both to sustain their relationship and to keep each of the partners active for as long as possible, were key elements of a 'nurturative relational context' and that it was a characteristic of couplehood rather than being an individual.

The third part of the study comprised a detailed analysis of the complete data set (n = 132 interviews) and allowed a more thorough understanding of the processes underpinning the 'nurturative relational context'. The analysis of this data found three temporally sequenced but overlapping phases: sustaining couplehood, maintaining involvement and becoming alone. Two of these phases often occurred simultaneously, though sustaining couplehood usually became more difficult and increasing effort was required in maintaining involvement. Eventually the non-affected spouse was left to become increasingly alone as the dementia progressed.

Making Sense and Adjusting to Loss

The idea of 'couplehood' has been further developed by Robinson et al. (2005) who collected data from couples comprising nine people with dementia and their family carers. The study found that the couples were involved in an ongoing process of 'making sense and adjusting to loss' and identified ten themes that developed in the interviews. These represented two higher order themes, 'Not the same person, tell me what is actually wrong' and 'Everything's changed, we have to go from here' (see Insert 6:1).

The first higher order theme described a cyclical process of gradually noticing changes in the person with dementia, and making

---

Insert 6:1 Themes relating to each of the two overriding themes Robinson et al. (2005)

Not the same person, tell me what is actually wrong

You don't notice straight away
Couples described a slow process of gradual realisation that the person with dementia was experiencing memory disorders.

Coming to the conclusion
As the process of realisation continued, many couples began to wonder about what might be happening. Couples described this as a shared process; with some couples talking together about the possibility that one person might have dementia.

I quite accepted it
Couples described a process of gradually accepting that one partner had dementia and that the memory problems were likely to be a permanent change in the person.

It did nothing for me
Couples described their dissatisfaction with the services they had experienced and the information they had received about dementia.

Coming here helped
Many couples described being supported by individual health professionals, despite their general dissatisfaction with the services offered. Partners found information more useful in helping them understand what was happening than did people with dementia.

Everything's changed, we have to go from here

I would say I have changed
Couples described progressive changes in the person with dementia over the period since they had received the diagnosis, focussing

Insert 6:1 cont'd

mainly on differences in memory functioning, mood and temperament. People with dementia talked about this time as being one in which they experienced feelings of depression, frustration and anxiety.

Taking over the reins
Couples described a difficult process of adjustment as the partner's role in the marital relationship changed as he or she in effect became a carer.

Take it as it comes
In spite of their difficulties, couples described a process of continuing their lives together as they always had and gradually adjusting together as a couple and as individuals.

Coping very well
Couples described a process of finding strategies to help them cope with their current difficulties as a couple and as individuals, which included the support they were receiving from other people.

I wouldn't mind doing it all again
Couples reminisced about their lives, generally talking about happier times as a couple and as individuals and comparing this to their current situation.

sense of the changes that occur as a couple, as well as couples' acceptance of their situation and their experiences of receiving a diagnosis. The second higher order theme described an oscillating process of acknowledging current difficulties and losses, and recognising resilience and developing coping strategies.

The work of Robinson et al. (2005) is helpful and contributes to our understanding of dyadic relationships that dementia care nurses encounter. However, caution should be exercised as the size of the sample in the study is quite small. However, it is curious that the study only seems to represent couples that have a good working relationship and is at odds with other studies such as that of Keady (1999) that finds that some couples have a poor relationship.

Triadic Approaches towards Dementia Care

Triadic approaches towards dementia care highlight the relationship between three people or agencies, typically the person with dementia, the primary informal carer, and with respect to dementia care nursing, the nurse.

Empirical work on triadic interaction in families initially arose in Family Therapy. Haley (1977) and Hoffman (1981) who identified the problematic nature of 'pathological triads' comprising three family members that often led to an alliance or collusion between two of these members and the exclusion of the third. This idea was applied to health care settings by Doherty and Baird (1983) who described the 'therapeutic triangle' between physicians, patients and the family.

Silliman (1989) initially developed a model of communication patterns in dementia care based on the idea of triadic interaction between the person with dementia, the informal carer and the health care professional. Studies on the triadic nature of interaction in nursing have been undertaken by Dalton (2003, 2005) and have been developed in relationship to dementia care by Adams (1999); Fortinsky (2001); Adams (2003) and Keady and Nolan (2003).

Early studies of triadic interaction examined the relationship between doctors, older people and their family carers (Haug, 1994; Hasselkus, 1994). Roscow (1981) and outlined how different coalitions can develop within triadic medical encounters that comprise the patient and the carer versus the doctor; the doctor and the carer versus the patient; and the doctor and the patient versus the carer. In the first coalition, it was argued that the alliance between the patient and the carer may limit the power of the doctor. In the second coalition, the coalition between doctor and the carer may challenge the patient and the patient's wishes may be ignored, dismissed or undermined. In the last coalition, the alliance between the doctor and the patient may outweigh the power possessed by the carer.

As a theoretical basis for this work, researchers drew on the work of the German sociologist Simmel (1964), who argued that the size of social groups affects their structure and functioning. Simmel identified three 'types' of role played by the third person within triads: the mediator, the exploiter, and the oppressor. Additional roles were developed by Caplow (1968) who outlined eight possible coalitions within three-person groups. Caplow argued further that coalitions develop as a result of members seeking to increase their own power and control within the triad.

The problematic nature of triadic interaction within service delivery has been noted by various writers. Biggs et al. (1995) highlight the collusive alliances that often develop and argue that 'the triangle of professional helper, carer and elder is thus the primary relation arising from community care' (p. 73). They suggest that

'[L]ike all triangular relationships it is inherently rivalrous, as there is always the possibility of two members pairing off, thus forming a collusive alliance that to some extent excludes the third party' (p. 73). Biggs (1993) proposes three types of collusive alliance. In the first, the informal carer and the professional helper exclude the older person. In the second, the informal carer and the older personally together ally against the professional helper. And in the third, the professional helper and the older person ally against the informal carer.

A similar understanding is shared by Twigg and Atkin (1994) who acknowledge the 'ambiguous position' (p. 11) of carers within community care. Twigg and Atkin (1994) outline various types of relationship between service agencies and carers that represent carers as acting either as resources, co-workers, co-clients or superseded carers, where a disabled person has no need of the carer. Twigg and Atkin (1994) argue that owing to their cognitive impairment, some people with dementia are unable to fully negotiate their own package of care and that some carers collude with their confused relative.

Relationship-centred Care and 'The Senses Framework'

Nolan et al. (2004) develop a model of triadic interaction, previously developed by Adams (1999); Fortinsky (2001) highlights the importance of interpersonal relationships in health and social care settings containing older people and describes it as 'relationship-centred care'. Through clearly influenced by person-centred care, relationship-centred care differs from person-centred care by adopting a triadic approach that includes the older person, the family carer and the paid-for carer, and highlights the reciprocal nature of communication between each participant.

An innovative aspect of relationship-centred care is that it highlights six 'Senses' which give rise to different subjective states within the older person, their carer and the paid-for carer. The six senses comprise: sense of security, continuity, belonging, purpose, achievement and significance (see Insert 6:2).

Shortcomings of Relationship-centred Care

Bearing in mind that relationship-centred care is 'still in construction', it has to be said that it contains a number of shortcomings. One shortcoming is that while relationship-centred care declares it goes 'beyond person-centred care' (Nolan et al., 2004), it also needs to go

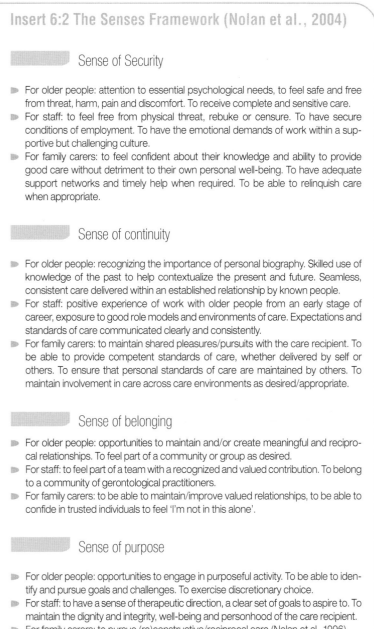

Insert 6:2 The Senses Framework (Nolan et al., 2004)

Sense of Security

- For older people: attention to essential psychological needs, to feel safe and free from threat, harm, pain and discomfort. To receive complete and sensitive care.
- For staff: to feel free from physical threat, rebuke or censure. To have secure conditions of employment. To have the emotional demands of work within a supportive but challenging culture.
- For family carers: to feel confident about their knowledge and ability to provide good care without detriment to their own personal well-being. To have adequate support networks and timely help when required. To be able to relinquish care when appropriate.

Sense of continuity

- For older people: recognizing the importance of personal biography. Skilled use of knowledge of the past to help contextualize the present and future. Seamless, consistent care delivered within an established relationship by known people.
- For staff: positive experience of work with older people from an early stage of career, exposure to good role models and environments of care. Expectations and standards of care communicated clearly and consistently.
- For family carers: to maintain shared pleasures/pursuits with the care recipient. To be able to provide competent standards of care, whether delivered by self or others. To ensure that personal standards of care are maintained by others. To maintain involvement in care across care environments as desired/appropriate.

Sense of belonging

- For older people: opportunities to maintain and/or create meaningful and reciprocal relationships. To feel part of a community or group as desired.
- For staff: to feel part of a team with a recognized and valued contribution. To belong to a community of gerontological practitioners.
- For family carers: to be able to maintain/improve valued relationships, to be able to confide in trusted individuals to feel 'I'm not in this alone'.

Sense of purpose

- For older people: opportunities to engage in purposeful activity. To be able to identify and pursue goals and challenges. To exercise discretionary choice.
- For staff: to have a sense of therapeutic direction, a clear set of goals to aspire to. To maintain the dignity and integrity, well-being and personhood of the care recipient.
- For family carers: to pursue (re)constructive/reciprocal care (Nolan et al., 1996).

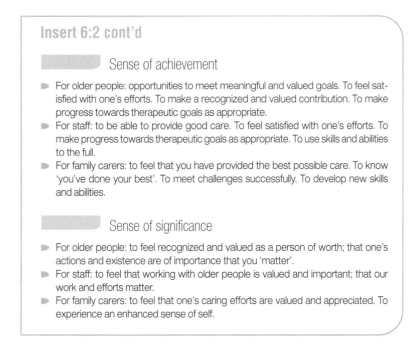

Insert 6:2 cont'd

Sense of achievement

- For older people: opportunities to meet meaningful and valued goals. To feel satisfied with one's efforts. To make a recognized and valued contribution. To make progress towards therapeutic goals as appropriate.
- For staff: to be able to provide good care. To feel satisfied with one's efforts. To make progress towards therapeutic goals as appropriate. To use skills and abilities to the full.
- For family carers: to feel that you have provided the best possible care. To know 'you've done your best'. To meet challenges successfully. To develop new skills and abilities.

Sense of significance

- For older people: to feel recognized and valued as a person of worth; that one's actions and existence are of importance that you 'matter'.
- For staff: to feel that working with older people is valued and important; that our work and efforts matter.
- For family carers: to feel that one's caring efforts are valued and appreciated. To experience an enhanced sense of self.

beyond person-centred care's use of symbolic interactionism and employ language-orientated approaches such as Conversation Analysis, Discourse Analysis and Narrative Analysis. A further shortcoming of relationship-centred care is that Nolan et al. (2004) fail to recognise that interaction within groups of three people is inherently problematic and often leads to the formation of coalitions and alliances between two triad members and the marginalisation of the third. The Senses Framework does not acknowledge what a lot of dementia care nurses know from their clinical experience that families caring for people with dementia often do not work together (Semple, 1992).

Systemic Approaches towards Dementia Care

A further concern about relationship-centred care and, indeed, person-centred care, is that each approach only highlights the informal carer *or* person with dementia. We would challenge this either/or way of thinking about dementia care that leads to the privilege and inclusion of one and the disadvantage and exclusion of the other. Instead, we would argue that people with dementia *and* their informal carers should each share an important place within dementia care nursing. Moreover, each approach forgets that different people and agencies outside the family contribute to people's experience of dementia. To address this, we would want to develop a whole systems approach towards dementia care nursing that while fully recognising the positive contribution of different approaches towards dementia care, such as person-centred care and relationship-centred care sees different people and agencies as contributing to the whole situation. We believe that this whole systems approach has much to offer dementia care nursing.

Moreover, the whole systems approach is able to accommodate recent advances in information technology and communication. In contemporary Western society, knowledge is no longer possessed only by elites such as the medical profession and is now available to the wider population, including people with dementia and their family members. This recent global phenomenon has been facilitated by the widespread use of the internet and has led to the creation of 'a network society' in which the flow of information between different agencies and participants in dementia care is more important than the position they have in society (Castells, 2000). Thus it is quite common for informal carers to know much more about dementia than some health care professionals and this may of course, challenge some professionals. In addition, the internet has led to the development of communities such as the Alzheimer's Society's Gay, Lesbian, Bisexual and Transvestite (GLBT) web site and numerous on-line discussion groups, in which knowledge is disseminated amongst its members and a sense of identity is shared. The rapid development of information technology has led to a clouding of the distinction between doctor/nurse and patient that was pervasive within the mental hospital and reflected the hierarchical nature of western society, and has given rise to the possibility of a more democratic form of dementia care. We see information technology as one way in which knowledge about people with dementia is disseminated, and links are made possible between different people and agencies, such as nursing homes, pressure groups and governmental bodies.

Knowledge is also shared through networks that are outside the internet through such methods as case conferences and telephone discussions between people with dementia, family members, nurses and different health and social care professionals. Communication in dementia care nursing people is much broader and more complex than suggested by person-centred care and triadic, relationship-centred care. Networking is a key phenomenon within dementia care nursing and occurs through interaction between many different individuals and through many different methods. While triadic approaches provide insights about communication between groups of three, dementia care nursing needs a much broader approach to capture its systemic nature.

We would draw on a broad-based systemic approach that captures the ongoing interrelationship between biological and social systems within dementia care nursing and draws upon Kitwood's dialectical understanding of the dementia process (Kitwood, 1997). As Rolland (1988) argues, 'the heart of all systems-orientated biopsychosocial inquiry is the focus on interaction' (p. 17). While we would suggest that insights developed by person-centred care and relationship-centred care contribute useful ways of seeing how people's identity and experience occur in dementia care nursing, we also believe that a broader systemic approach is required to recognise the contribution of wider systems, such as cultural and socio-political systems, upon the experience and identity of the person with dementia and their family.

The approach we adopt identifies the following systems:

- *Biological system*: within the person with dementia, their family members and paid-for carer(s).
- *Psychological system*: within the person with dementia, their family members and paid-for carer(s).
- *Family system*: concerned with roles, rules, boundary and the construction of family life.
- *Health and social care system*: includes all aspects of health and social care provision and includes the design of accommodation for older people with dementia, and financial aspects of their provision and its organisation.
- *Cultural system*: values, religious beliefs and customs possessed by different people involved with the provision of dementia care.
- *Socio-political system*: administration of health and social care for people with dementia and their carers.

The systemic nature of dementia care nursing corresponds well with the government document *Everybody's Business* (DH, 2005) and *Improving Services and Support for People with Dementia* (DH, 2007) which asserts that the care of older people with mental health conditions should be based on 'a whole systems approach'. In this approach, the care of people with dementia is seen in terms of the interdependency between the person with dementia, the family and other agencies. Carpenter and Treacher (1984) note that 'the family as a system should always be considered in terms of its interaction with other systems' (p. 4) and see systemic approaches as offering just as many insights into 'other systems', such as care organisations, as it does into the person and the family. Adopting a wider view is important when nursing people with dementia. Visits from the milkman, the postman and the home help all provide a systemic web of support that promotes the well-being of people with dementia and their informal carers. Systemic approaches have much to offer nurses working with people who have dementia and their families.

Systemic approaches have been developed by a long line of theorists (see Dallos and Draper, 2005). The work of Herr and Weakland (1979), Hargreave and Hanna (1997) and Curtis and Dixon (2005) have applied systems approaches to older people; Benbow et al. (1993), Fisher and Lieberman (1994), Garwick et al. (1994) and Szinovacz (2003) have applied them to people with dementia; and Friedman et al. (2003) and Wright and Leahey (2005) have applied them to nursing.

Systemic theory recognises that each family is unique and that family membership is affected by different systems, such as those relating to biological, legal, affectional, geographic and historical ties (Carr, 2000). These ideas are underpinned by General Systems Theory (Bertalanffy, 1968) and offer a way of understanding bio-psycho-medical phenomena, such as those nurses meet when working with people who have dementia. Underpinning systemic approaches are a number of ideas that include

- the importance of boundaries between different systems;
- the organization of sub-systems: for example, the person with dementia and their primary family carer is a sub-system of the family;
- the semi-permeability of boundaries: one system will affect another, for example, whatever is happening in the family system will affect what is happening in the system that constitutes the person with dementia – for example, when a carer is tired and irritated with a relative with dementia, it will affect what the person with dementia does and feels;

- the importance of patterns of inter-actions: what happens in one system will affect what happens in others;
- the acknowledgement that behaviour in systems is governed by rules (see Carr, 2000).

Systemic thinking has been applied to people with dementia, their family members and the wider community and is supported by the work of numerous academics, researchers and practitioners (Herr and Weakland, 1979; Gilleard, 1984; Niederehe and Fruge, 1984; Ratna and Davis, 1984; Woods et al., 1985; Benbow et al., 1993; Richardson et al., 1994; Marriott, 2000).

A systemic understanding of dementia care is outlined by Fisher and Lieberman (1994: p. 13) who argue that Alzheimer's disease has an impact upon spouses, offspring and in-laws and suggests that there is a need 'to broaden the scope of research and intervention with families of Alzheimer's disease'. Moreover, Szinovacz (2003) revealed the systemic effect of grandparents who have dementia, upon the relationship between parents and adolescents and argues that 'caregiving influences all family members, including adolescents exposed to the care situation' (p. 465) and found that 'caregiver's stress and family dynamics play an important role in the adaptation processes of family members, and that family integration may promote coping with the care situation, (p. 455).

Family Life Cycle and Dementia Care

An area of interest within systemic work concerns the family life cycle. This is the idea that over a period of time families pass through various developmental stages.

Carr (2000) identifies eight developmental tasks:

- those within the family of origin,
- leaving home,
- pre-marriage,
- childless couple,
- family with young children, family with adolescents,
- launching children and,
- later life.

Szinovacz (2003) found that while adolescents in families containing people with dementia frequently showed considerable empathy and respect for their parents acting as informal carers, they often complained about the spill-over of carer stress on to other relationships within the family, the focus of attention of their parents on care giving and lamented the restrictions placed on their own and their parents' activities. The importance of the family life cycle to nursing people with dementia is that many of the issues that arise in dementia care settings are due to the position of the family with respect to its place in the life cycle.

Approaches to Family Therapy and Dementia Care

Systemic work draws on a number of different theoretical approaches (Asen, 2004). Vetere and Dallos (2003) outline three approaches towards systemic work, all of which may be applied towards dementia care nursing. The first is concerned with understanding families in terms of their functions (Minuchin, 1974). The focus here is on the behaviour of family members, the development of boundaries between systems, and appropriate communication patterns. These ideas are helpful to dementia care nurses because they provide helpful insights into different issues associated with the care of the person with dementia (Mitrani et al., 2007). For example, they provide nurses with insights into who is 'in' the family and who is 'outside' that family and different conflicts that are encountered by family members within families in which someone has dementia, and who is talking and not talking to whom!

An important concept developed by Boss (2002) in her study of families containing people with dementia is 'family boundary ambiguity'. She understands this in terms of the degree of uncertainty among family members regarding who is in or who is out of the family and who is performing what roles and tasks within that system. She suggests that high family boundary ambiguity sets the stage for failing to cope with the stresses of giving care, and is often indicated by high levels of carer depression. She argues that when a person has dementia, that person is physically present in the family, though psychologically absent. This situation gives rise to family boundary ambiguity that is concerned with whether the person with dementia is actually inside or outside of the family. As with all forms of ambiguity, uncertainty occurs which often leads to carers experiencing stress and depression.

The second approach towards systemic work is the 'constructivist' approach which draws on developments in the social sciences in the 1970s and 1980s that highlight how people develop cognition, meaning and personal beliefs (Paré, 1995). Within this approach, people are seen in terms of what Vetere and Dallos (2003) call a 'personal biosphere' in which people construct their own understandings as they try to make sense of themselves and the world (Dallos, 1997). This approach offers nurses worthwhile insights into how social and interactive processes give rise to ways that various family members think about different situations. It might, for example, provide nurses with insights into how certain views and opinions that are possessed by certain family members may be contributing to the difficulties a family is experiencing caring for the person with dementia.

This approach has recently been developed by Keady et al. (2005), Williams and Keady (2004, 2006) who draw on life story work (Gubrium, 1993), constructivist grounded theory (Charmaz, 2000) and develop Co-constructed Inquiry (CCI). This innovative approach is concerned with enabling people who have dementia narrate and theorise about their experience using their own words (Williams and Keady, 2004, 2006), and argues that people's experience of dementia is co-constructed through the narratives and stories they encounter. They argue that people with dementia develop life histories that are influenced by such phenomena as previous exposure and lay understanding, ways of handling adverse life events, social and relational networks, coping patterns and so on. They argue that this approach is an effective way of working alongside people with dementia and their families and provides a sense of shared enterprise and discovery.

The third approach is 'social constructionism' (Burr, 2003). This approach is often confused with and used interchangeably with social constructivism (see Hughes et al., 2006: p. 24). However, Paré (p. 3) notes that '[C]onstructivism is primarily individualistic, focusing on sense data and information-processing rather than how language and other social practices organise the social order and people's position within it.' Underpinning this approach is the idea that 'human-systems are language-generating, meaning-generating systems engaged in an activity that is intersubjective and recursive' (Anderson and Goolishian, 1988: p. 5). This approach argues that people 'create the objects of our worlds with and through language' (p. 5) and that 'language does not mirror nature; language creates the natures we know. Meaning and understanding do not exist prior to the utterances of language' (p. 5) and that it is through communication that social reality is not only understood but also organised. Since dementia care nursing is primarily concerned with what nurses say and do, social constructionist approaches allow insights into how nurses shape dementia care settings and give rise to different participants having identity and position, obligation and responsibility and health and well-being. These phenomena do not exist in themselves and are mapped on to people and settings during the course of interactive and conversational exchanges within the dementia care setting. It is in this sense that dementia care nursing is socially constructed.

We would suggest that all these approaches towards systemic work help nurses understand social processes that occur in dementia care settings. Of these three approaches, the Critical Realist approach adopted in this book makes us more sympathetic to social constructivism and social constructionism. We would suggest that through these means people associated with the provision of dementia care nursing, including the person with dementia develop a sense of identity and selfhood (social constructivism) and their place within social groups and the wider social order (social constructionism).

Summary

To summarise, initially this chapter outlined various approaches that describe the interrelationship between the various people involved in the provision of dementia care. While the chapter identified insights that have been offered by dyadic and triadic approaches towards nursing people with dementia, it also revealed their shortcomings. To conclude, the chapter has outlined a whole systems approach towards dementia care nursing and has discussed its suitability as a meaning underpinning practice.

References

Adams, T. (1999). Developing partnership in dementia care: a discursive model of practice. In T. Adams and C. Clarke (eds). *Dementia Care: Developing Partnerships in Practice*. London: Baillière Tindall, pp. 37–56

Adams, T. (2003). Developing an inclusive approach to dementia care. *Practice* 15, 45–56.

Anderson, H. and Goolishian, H. A. (1988). Human systems as linguistic systems: preliminary and evolving ideas about the implications for clinical theory. *Family Process* 27, 4, 371–393.

Asen, E., Tomson, D., Young, V. and Tomson, P. (2004). *Ten Minutes for the Family*. London: Routledge.

Benbow, S., M. Marriott, A., Morley, M. and Walsh, S. (1993). Family therapy and dementia: review and clinical experience. *International Journal of Geriatric Psychiatry* 8, 717–725.

Bertalanffy, L. (1968). *General Systems Theory*. New York: Brazilier.

Biggs, S. (1993). User participation and interprofessional collaboration in community care. *Interprofessional Care* 7, 2, pp. 151–160.

Biggs, S., Phillipson, C. and Kingston, P. (1995). *Elder Abuse in Perspective*. Buckingham: Open University Press.

Boss, P. (2002) *Family Stress Management: A Contextual Approach*. (2nd ed.) London: Sage.

Burr, V. (2003). *Social Constructionism* (2nd ed.). London: Routledge.

Caplow, T. (1968). *Two against One: Coalitions in Triads*. Englewood Cliffs: Prentice Hall.

Carpenter, J. and Treacher, A. (1983). (eds). *Using Family Therapy*. London: Blackwell.

Carpenter, J. and Treacher, A. (1984). Introduction: using family therapy. In A. Treacher and J. Carpenter, (eds). *Using Family Therapy*. Oxford: Basil Blackwell.

Carr, A. (2000). *Family Therapy: Concepts, Processes and Practice*. Wiley: Chichester.

Castells, M. (2000). *The Rise of the Network Society*. (2nd ed.) Oxford: Blackwell.

Charmaz, K. (2000). Grounded theory: objectivist and constructivist methods. In N. K. Denzin and T. S. Lincoln (eds). *Handbook of Qualitative Research*. (2nd ed.). Thousands Oaks, CA: Sage, pp. 509–535.

Curtis, E. A. and Dixon, M. S. (2005). Family therapy and systemic practice with older people: where are we now? *Journal of Family Therapy* 27, 43–64.

Dallos, R. (1997). *Interacting Stories: Narratives, Family Beliefs and Therapy*. London: Karnac Books.

Dallos, R. and Draper, R. (2005). *An Introduction to Family Therapy: Systemic Theory and Practice* (2nd ed.) Maidenhead: Open University Press.

Dalton, J. M. (2003). Development and testing of the theory of collaborative decision-making in nursing practice for triads. *Journal of Advanced Nursing* 41, 1, 22–33.

Dalton, J. M. (2005). Client-caregiver-nurse formation in decision-making situations during home visits. *Journal of Advanced Nursing* 52, 3, 291–299.

Department of Health (1999). *The Carer's National Strategy*. London: The Stationary Office.

Department of Health (2005). *Everybody's Business: Integrated Mental Health Services for Older Adults. A Service Development Guide*. London: Care Services Improvement Partnership (CSIP).

Department of Health (2006). *A New Ambition for Old Age: Next Steps in Implementing the National Service Framework for Older People*. London: Department of Health.

Department of Health (2006). *From Values to Action: The Chief Nursing Officer's Review of Mental Health Nursing*. London: Department of Health.

Department of Health (2007). *Improving Services and Support for People with Dementia*. London: TSO.

Doherty, W. J. and Baird, M. A. (1983). *Family Therapy and Family Medicine: Toward the Primary Care of Families*. New York: Guilford Press.

Fisher, L. and Lieberman, M. A. (1994). Alzheimer's disease: the impact of the family on spouses, offspring, and inlaws. *Family Process* 33, 305–325.

Fortinsky, R. H. (2001). Health care triads and dementia care: Integrative frameworks and future directions. *Aging and Mental Health* 5, 2, S1, 35–48.

Friedman, M., Bowden, V. R. and Jones, E. (2003). *Family Nursing: Research, Theory and Practice 5th Edition*. New Jersey: Prentice Hall.

Garwick, A. W., Detzner, D. and Boss, P. (1994). Family perceptions of living with Alzheimer's disease. *Family Process* 33, 327–340.

Gilleard, C. (1984). *Living with Dementia*. Beckenham: Croom Helm.

Gubrium, J. R. (1993). *Speaking of Life: Horizons of Meaning for Nursing Home Residents*. Newbury Park, CA: Sage.

Haley, J. (1977). Toward a system of psychological systems. In P. Watzlawick and J. Weakland (eds) *The Interactional View*. New York: Norton.

Hargrave, T. D. and Hanna, S. M. (eds) (1997). *The Aging Family: New Visions in Theory, Practice and Reality*. New York: Brunner/Mazel.

Hasselkus, B. R. (1994). Three-track care: Patient, family member and physician in the medical visit. *Journal of Aging Studies* 8, 3, 291–307.

Haug, M. R. (1994). Elderly patients, caregivers, and physicians: Theory and research on health care triads. *Journal of Health and Social Behaviour* 35, 1, 1–12.

Helleström, I. (2005). *Explored 'Couplehood' in Dementia: A Constructivist Grounded Theory Study*. Dissertation in submission to PhD. Sweden: Institute for the Study of Later Life, Linköping University.

Helleström, I., Nolan, M. and Lundh, U. (2005a). We do things together. *Dementia: The International Journal of Social Research and Practice* 4, 1, 7–22.

Helleström, I., Nolan, M. and Lundh, U. (2005b). Awareness context theory and the dynamics of dementia. *Dementia: The International Journal of Social Research and Practice* 4, 2, 269–295.

Herr, J. J. and Weakland, J. H. (1979). *Counselling Elders and their Families: Practical Techniques for Applied Gerontology.* New York: Springer.

Hoffmann, L. (1981). *Foundations of Family Therapy.* New York: Basic Books.

Hughes, J., Louw, S. J. and Sabat, S. (2006). Seeing whole. In J. C. Hughes, S. J. Louw and S. R. Sabat (eds) *Dementia: Mind, Meaning and the Person.* Oxford: Oxford University Press, pp. 1–39.

Hutchinson, S. A., Leger-Krall, S. and Wilson, H. S. (1997). Early probably Alzheimer's disease and awareness context theory. *Social Science and Medicine* 45, 9, 1399–1409.

Keady, J. (1999). *The Dynamics of Dementia: A Modified Grounded Theory Study.* PhD Thesis, Bangor: University of Wales.

Keady, J. and Nolan, M. (2003). The dynamics of dementia: working together, working separately, or working alone. In M. Nolan, U. Lunth, G. Grant and J. Keady (eds) *Partnerships in Family Care: Understanding the Caregiving Carer.* Buckingham: Open University Press, pp. 15–32.

Keady, J., Williams, S. and Hughes-Roberts, J. (2005). Emancipatory practice development through life-story work: Changing care in a memory clinic in North Wales. *Practice Developments in Health Care* 4, 4, 202–212.

Kitwood, T. (1997). *Dementia Reconsidered.* Buckingham: Open University Press.

Marriott, A. (2000). *Family Therapy with Older Adults and their Families.* Bicester: Speechmark.

Minuchin, S. (1974). *Families and Family Therapy.* Cambridge, MA: Harvard University Press,

Mitrani, V., Lewis, J., Feaster, D., Czaja, S., Eisdorfer, C., Schulz, R. and Szapocznik, J. (2007). The Role of Family Functioning in the Stress Process of Dementia Caregivers: A Structural Family Framework. *The Gerontologist* 46, 97–105.

Niederehe, G. and Fruge, E. D. (1984). Dementia and family dynamics: clinical research issues. *Journal of Geriatric Psychiatry* 17, 1, 21–60.

Nolan, M. R., Grant, G. and Keady, J. (1996). *Understanding Family Care: A Multi-Disciplinary Model of Caring and Coping.* Buckingham: Open University Press.

Nolan, M., Ryan, T., Enderby, P. and Reid, D. (2002). Towards a more inclusive vision of dementia care practice. *Dementia: The International Journal of Social Research and Practice* 1, 2, 193–211.

Nolan, M. R., Davies, S., Brown, J., Keady, J. and Nolan J. (2004). Beyond 'person-centred' care: a new vision for gerontological nursing. *Journal of Clinical Nursing* 13, s1, 45–53.

Paré, D. (1995). Of families and other cultures: The shifting paradigm of family therapy. *Family Process* 34, 1–20.

Ratna, L. and Davis, L (1984). Family therapy with the elderly mentally ill. Some strategies and techniques. *The British Journal of Psychiatry* 145, 311–315.

Richardson, C. A., Gilleard, C. J., Lieberman, S. and Peelerg, R. (1994). Working with older adults and their families – a review. *Journal of Family Therapy* 16, 225–240

Robinson, L., Clare, L. and Evans, K. (2005). Making sense of dementia and adjusting to loss: Psychological reactions to a diagnosis of dementia in couples. *Aging and Mental Health* 9, 4, 337–347.

Rolland, J. S. (1988). A conceptual model of chronic and life-threatening illness and its impact. In S. Chilman, E. W. Nunnally and F Cox. (eds) *Chronic Illness and disability. The Trouble with Families.* Vol. 2. London: Sage, pp. 17–68.

Roscow, I. (1981). Coalitions in geriatric medicine. In M. R. Haug (ed) *Elderly Patients and their Doctors.* New York: Springer. pp. 137–146.

Scottish Executive (2006). *Rights, Relationships and Recovery.* Edinburgh: Scottish Executive.

Semple, S. (1992). Conflict in Alzheimer's caregiving families: its dimensions and consequences. *Gerontologist* 32, 5, 648–655.

Silliman, R. A. (1989). Caring for the frail older patient: The doctor-patient-caregiver relationship. *Journal of General Internal Medicine* 4, 237–241.

Simmel, G. (1964). The dyad and the triad. In L. A. Coser and B. Rosenberg (eds) *Sociological Theory: A Book of Readings.* New York: The Macmillan Company.

Szinovacz, M. E. (2003). Caring for a demented relative at home: effects on parent-adolescent relationships and family dynamics. Journal of Aging Studies 17, 445–472.

Twigg, J. A. and Atkin, K. (1994). Carers: Perceived: Policy and Practice in Informal Care. Buckingham: Open University Press.

Vetere, A. and Dallos, R. (2003). *Working Systemically with Families: Formulation, Intervention and Evaluation.* London: Karnac.

Williams, S. and Keady, J. (2004). Writing Lives: the development of nurse education by using the biographies of older people – a reflective account. In D. Robinson, C. Horrocks, N. Kelly, and B. Roberts (eds). *Narrative, Memory and Identity: Theoretical and Methodological Issues.* Huddersfield: University of Huddersfield Press. pp. 193–200.

Williams, S. and Keady, J. (2006) Editorial: the narrative voice of people with dementia. *Dementia* 5, 163–166.

Woods, A., Niederehe, G. and Frugé, E. (1985). Dementia: A family System Perspective. *Generations* 10, 1, 19–23.

Wright, L. M. and Leahey, M. (2005). *Nurses and Families: A guide to family assessment and intervention.* (4th ed.) Philadelphia, PA: F.A. Davis Company.

Chapter 7

Assessment and care planning within dementia care nursing

Trevor Adams

Learning Outcomes

After reading the chapter you will be able to

- describe what is meant by 'nursing assessment' and 'care planning' within dementia care nursing;
- describe the difference between multi-agency and professional assessment in how nursing assessments and care planning give rise to the social construction of situations within dementia care nursing;
- discuss the issue of risk and its implication for assessment and care planning when nursing people with dementia and their families;
- critically describe different principles associated with recording nursing assessments.

Introduction

The previous chapters have outlined the historical and socio-political background to dementia care nursing, a critique of existing medical, person-centred and relationship-centred approaches towards dementia care and have put forward a whole systems approach towards dementia care nursing. This present chapter uses this approach as a guide to the assessment of dementia care settings and the planning of care within dementia care nursing. Underpinning the approach taken in this chapter are those ideas developed in Chapter 6, and believe that the whole systems approach should shape how dementia care nurses undertake each part of the nursing process, including assessment and care planning.

What Is Assessment within Dementia Care Nursing?

Assessment is the first stage of the nursing process that comprises assessment, planning, intervention and evaluation. Barker (1997) views nursing assessments as decision-making processes that are based on the collection of relevant information, using a formal set of ethical criteria, which contribute to the overall evaluation of the person and their situation. This way of understanding nursing assessments focus on its outcomes. While outcomes are certainly an important aspect of nursing assessments, we would also want to highlight the process of assessment and the opportunity to learn more about the person with dementia and their family.

Nursing and Multi-agency Assessments

Two types of assessment occur in dementia care nursing: multi-agency and professional assessment. Multi-agency assessment is concerned with implementing a single, shared approach towards assessment. Professional assessments, however, are assessments undertaken by a particular profession such as the medical profession or the nursing profession. At the present time, social policy does not offer one approach towards assessing people with dementia and their family members. *Everybody's Business* describes two approaches that presently exist in relationship towards assessment: the Single Assessment Process (DH, 2001) and the Care Programme Approach (CPA) (DH, 2006). The situation is confusing, and it is not surprising that *Everybody's Business* (DH, 2005) says that the Department of Health is considering developing one assessment tool for use with all people who have complex needs. *Everybody's Business* outlines various key messages about assessment within services for older people with mental health conditions:

- services should place the user at the centre of assessment and care planning. The service user's views of their own abilities and desired outcomes should be central to the process;
- services should aim to improve standards of assessment and care planning with a common method across agencies and care settings;
- the CPA and Single Assessment Process are frameworks that offer a multi-disciplinary/multi-agency working, which help co-ordinate the roles and responsibilities of different professionals across health, social care and other appropriate organisations;
- the level and type of assessment should be proportionate to need, and information should be shared and built on; and,

▶ may differ significantly from those of the user but the same principles should apply (DH, 2005: p. 15).

Undertaking Nursing Assessments of People with Dementia and Their Families

In the previous chapters, we argued that nurses working with people who have dementia should adopt a dialectical approach in which people's experience of dementia, is seen to arise out of the ongoing interrelationship between biological and social systems within dementia care situations (Kitwood, 1997). In addition we have suggested that a Critical Realist approach lends its support towards constructionist approaches that understand dementia care nursing in terms of what nurses do and say that give rise to a particular way in which dementia care situations are understood and organised. This understanding of dementia care nursing may be applied to how nurses should undertake assessments with people who have dementia and their families, with specific reference to what nurses should say and do.

Often assessments are concerned with finding out what other people cannot do, rather than about what they can do. We would argue that often nurses undertaking assessments allow the person with dementia and their informal carers to feel bad about themselves and gain a negative impression of what they can do to promote their own and other people's well-being.

We would therefore support a 'strengths' approach towards nursing assessment in dementia care nursing. Rather than seeing people's difficulties and weaknesses, we believe that it is much more productive to see what the person with dementia and their family members *can do* and use this assessment to build their personal and social resources to optimise their well-being. *Rights, Relationships and Recovery* (Scottish Executive, 2006) advocates a strengths model of case management in which assessment is a crucial part. This model may be adapted for use within dementia care nursing (Insert 7:1).

However, it is not just how people see themselves that arise within assessments, the way different clinical situations are viewed also arises within assessments such as people's needs, concerns and responsibilities and as we will see later in the chapter, how certain situations are seen as a risk.

Insert 7:1 The 'strengths' model of case management applied to dementia care nursing

▶ Focus on strengths of people with dementia and their family carers rather than their deficits.

▶ The community is viewed as an 'oasis' of resources – the emphasis is on engaging people in existing community services rather than specialist dementia care services.

▶ Interventions are based on the principles of allowing the person with dementia maximum information about services and optimal choice.

▶ The nurse/person with dementia/family carer relationship is primary and essential.

▶ Dementia care nurses should visit people with dementia and their family members in their own or preferred environments.

▶ People with dementia and their family carers have the ability to continue to grow, learn and change.

In nursing assessments in dementia care nursing, different people and agencies are involved and each will have their own views and opinions about what is happening in the dementia care setting. Nursing assessments need to capture these views and allow different people to have their say and fully describe what has happened, what is happening and what should happen. In this pluralistic and inclusive understanding of assessment, any attempt by one person to take over the assessment and exclude the views of the others should be challenged by the nurse. It is important to recognise that nursing assessments are not politically neutral, and that everybody should as far as possible, have a chance to put forward their views (Taylor and White, 2000).

We would also suggest that there is a degree of subjectivity and interpretation in all nursing assessments and that they should not be seen simply as a means of 'getting the facts'. In line with the Critical Realist approach adopted in this book, we would argue that different accounts and stories in dementia care settings are given by different people at different times. When this happens nurses have to decide how they can best represent each version of events. Thus, there is a rhetorical edge to nursing assessments as accounts given by people with dementia, family members and different health and social care professionals, will put forward their version of events (Billig, 1987).

This may best be seen by looking at a situation in which you were assessed, say, when you were last interviewed for a job. While you would not have wanted to tell the interviewers a lie, you probably would have been careful about exactly what you said. No doubt you took care not to reveal anything that might cast you in a bad light with the interviewers. This may have meant not telling the interviewers the full story about everything and that some of the answers you gave were tailored to what you thought they might want to hear. You would, hopefully, have been able to tell the interviewers all the good things about you in the hope that they might offer you the job. Overall, you probably took great care to make sure the interviewer got a good impression of you so that you got what you wanted – the job!

In the same way, nursing assessments should be seen as a time when people with dementia and different family carers all have their own, sometimes competing, views and agendas, and through the use of accounts and stories attempt to influence decision-making and what eventually might happen. This is not to suggest that people are devious and underhanded but rather that what is said and done in nursing assessments socially constructs people and situations and gives rise to a particular way the dementia care setting is viewed and organised. Nursing assessments offer people the opportunity to provide an account of what is happening, identify particular people who are involved in the provision of care and put forward particular decisions about future care. What is of particular concern is that people with dementia, as a result of cognitive impairment, are often much less able to contribute towards the representation of dementia care settings within nursing assessments and will often find themselves overwhelmed by other people's ability to make their views known. Indeed, Keady and Bender (1998) argue that the process of assessment itself could subordinate the person with dementia, and make them worry about whether they might be moved out of their own home and placed into a care home, and so further lose their ability to make their own choices.

People with dementia may experience within nursing assessments excess disability, as they are treated as more disabled than they actually are. Nichols et al. (1998) argue that people who are diagnosed as having dementia are often seen to have poor judgement and difficulty when making decisions. However, Feinberg and Whitlach (2001) suggest that people with mild to moderate cognitive impairment are quite able to provide constant responses to questions about themselves, their preferences and choices. In a study investigating the ability of 88 older adults with mild to moderate dementia to give informed medical consent, Moye et al. (2004) found that although people with dementia did experience limitations in their understanding of treatment and information concerning their treatment, most were considered legally competent to make decisions. It is for such reasons that good practice in assessment should allow nurses to adopt a strengths approach that hears the voice of the person with dementia and helps them to express their own views and opinions.

Who Should Be Assessed?

Three forms of assessments are used in dementia care:

- assessment of the person with dementia;
- assessment of the family carer(s);
- assessment of how the person with dementia and their family carer(s) work together.

Each of these contributes important information that may be used to plan care. While the assessment of either the person with dementia or their family carer(s) alone offers a simple and brief assessment of the situation, it is likely to be one-sided and represent the views of only one person.

Nursing assessments of people with dementia can take place in a range of clinical settings, at various stages of the dementia. Usually a nursing assessment of someone with dementia and their relatives occurs over a period of time (Marrelli, 2005). There are a number of reasons why a nursing assessment should not just gain information at just one point of time, for example, the person with dementia may have a short physical illness and also, one visit may not be enough to gather the vast amount of information that is available. Moreover, it often takes a number of visits for a person with dementia and their family carer(s) to feel comfortable and open up and talk about personal and, sometimes, intimate areas of their life. It is therefore probably best to think of a nursing assessment as an ongoing process that occurs at the same time as other parts of the nursing process, such as care planning, implementation and evaluation.

As we have already discussed, a good nursing assessment will represent people in terms of what they can do. These areas may then be addressed in the nursing care plan and provide a means of enhancing the well-being of the person with dementia or their family carer(s).

Information may be gained in the nursing assessment by three methods.

▶ *Semi-structured interviews* in which the nurse asks questions such as 'How have you been feeling lately' or 'What do you like about going to Day Care?' This approach is exploratory and allows the person with dementia and their family members to tell their own story, while at the same time allowing discussion on other issues that are relevant to the dementia care setting.

▶ *Questionnaires and rating scales* are sometimes used in assessments in dementia care nursing and are usually directed towards one specific clinical area. Sayers (2005) identifies a number of questionnaires and rating scales that are used within nursing assessments in dementia care: Mini Mental Status Examination (MMSE) (Folstein et al., 1975); Cambridge Mental Disorder of the Elderly (CAMDEX) (Brayne and Calloway, 1989); and the Care Giver Strain Questionnaire (Robinson, 1983). In particular clinical situations, such as memory clinics, a more extensive range of tests may be used (Adams and Page, 2000).

▶ *Direct observation* is also an important source of information that is used by dementia care nurses during assessments and may take the form of information gained by the nurses by sight (colour of skin or facial expression), hearing (listening to what the person with dementia says) and smell (urine or faecal odour as an indication of possible incontinence).

Barker (2003: p. 75) outlines various stages within a nursing assessment: in the initial stage, information is mainly gained from unstructured interviews, rather than focusing on more specific and detailed issues. However, as the assessment proceeds, information is gained from more detailed examination of issues identified earlier in the assessment. It is important to realise that a good assessment will rely on the information gained from natural conversations rather than those that arise from an externally introduced interview schedule. Barker et al. (2003: p. 64) says that there is an 'ordinariness' about nursing assessments that is characterised by participants sharing stories about what is happening.

Care Planning

A nursing care plan is based on the ongoing assessment and comprises an outline of actions which the person with dementia, the family members or the nurse will do to address various issues that are considered problematic and that will undermine the well-being of the person with dementia and their family members. We believe that all care plans are tentative and that following the full collaboration, negotiation and agreement of everyone involved in the dementia care setting – including the person with dementia – a nursing care plan may be changed and amended. We, thus, would support the shared ownership of the nursing care plan by the nurse, the person with dementia and the family carer(s). Typically, the care plan should contain a statement of the goals that have been agreed, a description of any actions to be taken and specified criteria against which an evaluation of progress can be made. Ryrie and Norman (2004: p. 203) argue that the care plan should contain various 'goal statements' and that these statements should be characterised by the acronym SMART: Specific, Measurable, Achievable, Realistic and Time Limited. Moreover, care plans should be under continual review and should be updated as soon as an intervention has been attempted. It is important to have a written copy of the care plan as this is a source of evidence of professional practice; an updated copy of the care plan is also helpful to the person with dementia and other family members as this will increase their sense of joint participation. It may well be appropriate for other health and social care professionals also to have a copy of the nursing care plan.

Risk, Assessment and Care Planning in Dementia Care Nursing

The assessment of risk is an important aspect of nursing assessments. There has been considerable concern about identifying and responding to risk within dementia care settings, and we would like to address this issue by developing an understanding that corresponds to the Critical Realist approach adopted by the book. Studies on the assessment of risk in health care settings have usually viewed risk in naïve realist terms, and see risks as occurring 'out there' and having an existence that is independent of people. In this way, a risk is a risk whatever anybody thinks about it. We would, however, want to adopt a critical rather than naïve form of realism

in which the risk has an objective existence but its meaning is negotiated by social and conversational processes, by what people do
and say. The implications of this approach is that first, nurses are not
the only people who characterise different situations as risky.
Second, people with dementia contribute to particular circumstances being seen as a risk and that their view should be heard. And
third, risk should not always be avoided but rather should be considered within the decision-making process.

While the possibility that people with dementia and their
families may place themselves in risky situations should be taken
seriously, thinking and acting as though people with dementia and
their informal carers are unable to make these decisions for themselves is infantilising and promotes a restrictive form of nursing
which is perhaps more concerned with protecting the interests of the
nurse rather than the person with dementia (Manthorpe, 2004). Risk
is a part of everybody's daily life and there is a need for dementia
care nurses to recognise that not only do certain situations pose a
risk but also that some risks are reasonable to take. We therefore
think that decisions about risky situations should be made between
people with dementia, family carer(s) and relevant health and social
care practitioners and thus, we would adopt a whole systems
approach. Within this approach, we would see dementia care nurses
eliciting the views and opinions of the person with dementia and
their family members, facilitating discussion about the possibility of
risk, offering additional knowledge and experience, and helping the
person with dementia develop 'low risk' care plans that enable them
to carry out their wishes.

Morgan and Wetherell (2004) develop the idea of 'positive risk-
taking' and argue that people can only grow and develop through
measured and justified risk taking. They would also add that risk-
taking should be intelligent and negotiated between the user and
carer(s). While the idea of positive risk-taking has developed in
services for younger people, we would argue that it is just as
applicable with older people who have dementia and their family
members.

Risk to Self

Clarke and Heyman (1999) and Clarke (2000) highlight that different
people may have different views on what constitutes a risk in dementia care and distinguish between the professional's views on risk and

that of family members. They argue that professional views are often based on a pathological model of dementia and are closely associated with the inevitability of physical and mental decline. They found family carers saw situations very differently, and tended to see things in more specific ways which focused on the person with dementia. They recommend that professionals should listen to the views of family carers on what constitutes a risk in particular situations.

More recently, the way risk is negotiated between people with dementia, family members and nurses has been examined. My own study (Adams, 2001) found that community mental health nurses (CMHN) and family carers frequently co-construct situations as 'risky' through the course of four stages:

Stage 1: Fishing

The first stage is 'fishing' in which the CMHN raised issues that allowed the family carer the opportunity to raise any issues that may be considered as a risk (See Extract 1).

Extract 1

1. CMHN: How do you feel about
2.   your mum in the last three
3.   weeks since we met?
4. Mrs Hayes: She I think she's deteriorated
5.   I think quite rapidly actually.

This is a frequent pattern of interaction in meetings between CMHNs and family members and consists of the CMHN making an utterance (Extract 1 lines 1–3) which introduces a subject area. As a result of the dominance of professionals within meetings with 'lay' members, fishing is usually initiated by the CMHN. In Extract 2, the CMHN asks the carer about his own personal well-being, which he says is 'not too bad' (line 2). This comment is ambiguous and the CMHN fishes again and asks whether 'things have been difficult' (line 4) and allows the carer to say that things have been difficult (lines 5–6). The CMHN allows the carer to infer that he takes Mr Stott's difficulties seriously by saying 'Really' (line 7).

Extract 2

1. CMHN: How are you?
2. Mr Stott: Not too bad.

3. CMHN:　　Are you sure? Ha'
4.　　　　　things been difficult?
5. Mr Stott:　Yeh about the last two or
6.　　　　　three days particularly.
7. CMHN:　　Really

Stage 2: Risk Identification
'Risk identification' occurs as a result of fishing and comprises utterances made by the carer that allow the inference that a particular situation is a risk. In Extract 1 as a result of the CHMN's question, the carer says 'I think quite rapidly actually' (lines 5) and also in Extract 2 when Mr Stott says that things have been difficult in 'the last two or three days particularly' (lines 5–6).

Another strategy used in risk identification is for the CMHN to seize upon something that a carer is saying in the meeting.

Extract 3
1. CPN:　　　So do you think Alice is losing weight?
2. Mr Jacobs:　Doesn't seem to.
3. CMHN:　　　Clothes don't seem extra big or falling off her?
4. Mr Jacobs:　No, no, no.
5. CMHN:　　　Have you...?
6. Mr Jacobs:　The sherry keeps that up.
7. CMHN:　　　O:::::r the sherry?
8. Mr Jacobs:　She likes sherry
9. CMHN:　　　Does she? What a lot?
10. Mr Jacobs:　Quite a lot.

Extract 3 shows the CMHN fishing by asking Mr Jacobs if his wife is losing weight (line 1). The carer says that he does not think she is losing weight (line 2) and thus, does not consider weight loss as a risk. This understanding is affirmed by the CMHN saying that her '[C]lothes don't seem extra big or falling off her' (line 3) and thus, displays its co-construction. In line 5, the CMHN is interrupted when Mr Jacobs says 'The sherry keeps that up' (line 6). The CMHN highlights 'the sherry' in line 7 and asks Mr Jacobs two questions about his wife's drinking habits (line 9). The inference that Alice's sherry drinking might constitute a risk is inferred from Mr Jacobs' comments that his wife drinks sherry and likes it.

Stage 3: Risk Assessment
CMHN then usually asks further questions to gain a more complete description of the situation before creating, if necessary, an action plan.

Extract 4

1.	Mrs Jones:	… and every evening she says 'Oh I must
2.		go now', 'I've got to get the children', or 'The children
3.		will be home' or 'They've got to go to school in
4.		the morning', you know, because this happens nearly
5.		every night. And I think it happens more because she's
6.		had the drink.
7.	CMHN:	Right
8.	Mrs Jones:	Well, I, she'd most probably ask those things
9.		but the more it goes on and on, I think.
10.	CMHN:	Yes, how much she is having to drink then?
11.	Mrs Jones:	Well, you see to somebody really
12.		alright she likes two drinks, well she likes
13.		three and I try to spread them Mind they're are not very big.
14.	CMHN:	No. Yes.
15.	Mrs Jones:	But, yes. And she wants to have three, well
16.		the more she has the more she wants
17.		and I try to, I keep it to three and no more
18.		that's definitely it, you know.
19.	CMHN:	Yes.
20.	Mrs Jones:	Because as soon as she's had one drink
21.		things start to go a bit haywire, more so
22.		you know.

In Extract 4, the CMHN makes utterances (lines 10, 14 and 19) and that allow Mrs Jones to infer that the CMHN would like to know more about a particular issue – again, the drinking habits of a relative with dementia. Mrs Jones accepts this invitation (lines 11–13, 15–18 and 20–22).

At this point, the CMHNs may decide to take no further action, address the risk outside the meeting or attempt to manage the situation in the meeting with the family carer.

Stage 4: Risk Management
This occurs if the nurse decides to take an action to reduce the risk that has been constructed within the interview (see Insert 7:2).

Insert 7:2 Case Example

Mrs Andrews had moderate dementia and spent nearly every day of the week going on buses to all the local and not so local markets in Ashton, Bury, Rochdale and Stockport. This is what she had always done throughout her life and, indeed, was her life. It was quite easy to imagine (particularly when lying in bed at 3 o'clock in the morning!) that she might get lost or run over by a car. But she never did. The CMHN and other members of the multi-disciplinary team felt that it would be totally inappropriate and quite impractical to stop this woman from making these daily journeys. While the team still thought there was a risk, it was decided that we, including the woman herself, should live with the risk and that, at least for the time being, she should be allowed to visit the markets.

Sometimes, though, the risk is too great and out of keeping with what society is willing to accept. I once was working with a man who was in the early stages of dementia who was living alone and who liked 'Do-It-Yourself'. On one occasion, the man was found, or at least it was said he was (!) taking an electric socket out of the wall while the electricity was still turned on. Accounts of this incident raised considerable concern amongst many of the health and social care workers involved in the case. It was decided that the man was too much a risk to live on his own and it was decided to move him to a more suitable type of accommodation, where he was not so likely to electrocute himself. This was against his will, though the argument was that it was in his best interests, and for that matter those of his neighbours!

While this approach is helpful, it does leave some uneasy questions unanswered. Look at the last example. How do we really know what happened? How do we know that the man nearly electrocuted himself? What did he say he was doing? As the story got hyped up, were things added to it? Who was likely to benefit from the story? The point is that none of the health and care workers had actually seen what had happened and had only heard the story from the neighbours who may have been worried about what might eventually happen. The only way we knew about it was through stories told by those involved in the situation. Having an interest in the situation allows the possibility that what one speaker says had happened might be tailored to getting a particular outcome. This makes sense when it is remembered that health and social care workers may be seen by family members and neighbours as having access to much sought after resources such as day care and residential care.

In another case, I was told that an old lady I was visiting had repeatedly seen a leading television personality come out of her television set and walk around her living room. She was not at all distressed by this. The only person who was upset was her son-in-law, who was concerned that his wife was spending too much time with her mother. He wanted and argued forcibly that his mother-in-law should go into a residential home. The old lady did not see herself as being at risk, and neither did I. After talking to the old lady and the other members of her family, I came to the conclusion that the risk to the old lady was something that was merely constructed by what her son-in-law was saying, and that his interests and agenda were not the same as those of either the person with dementia or her daughter.

An associated problem is that the mere possibility that there is a risk poses a threat to the nurse. If the risk happens, not only will the person with dementia incur its consequences, the nurse themselves could well be seen as negligent and incompetent. Thus, there is always a tendency for nurses to insure themselves and prevent the possibility that their reputation may eventually become tarnished.

Good Record Keeping

An important part of assessment and care planning is writing it up. This is very important as not only will it promote communication between different members of the multi-disciplinary team, but it will also provide a source of evidence. This is very important in an increasingly litigious society and it is very important that nurses can provide written evidence that they have undertaken certain nursing actions. Various suggestions can be made about how nurses may enhance the quality of their records (see Insert 7:3).

Insert 7:3 Guidance for good record keeping in dementia care nursing

- Record keeping is an integral part of nursing people with dementia.
- Good records are a mark of a skilled and safe nurse.

Insert 7:3 cont'd

- Records should not use abbreviations, jargon, meaningless phrases, irrelevant speculation or offensive subjective comments about people with dementia or family carers.
- Records should be written in a way that the family members should be able to understand.
- By auditing your records, you can assess the standard of the records and identify areas for improvement and staff development.
- You must ensure that any entry in a record can be easily identified.
- Patients and clients have the right of access to records that are held about them.
- Each practitioner's contribution to records should be seen as of equal importance.
- You have a duty to protect the confidentiality of the person with dementia and their records.
- People with dementia should own their healthcare records, as far as it is possible to do so and as long as they're happy to do so.
- The principle of confidentiality of information held about the people with dementia is just as important in relation to computer-held records as for all other records.
- The use of records in research should be approved by local research ethics committees.
- You must use your professional judgement to decide what is relevant and what should be recorded.
- Records must be clearly written and in such a manner that the text cannot be erased.
- Records should be factual, consistent and accurate.
- You should assume that any entry you make will be scrutinised at a later date.
- Good record keeping protects the welfare of people with dementia.

Summary

This chapter examines the nature of nursing assessments and describes how nursing assessments and care plans may be undertaken within dementia care nursing. The chapter identifies two forms of assessment – multi-disciplinary agency assessment and professional assessment. Underpinning the chapter is the view that nurses should adopt a 'strengths approach' towards assessments that acknowledges and reinforces the abilities of the person with dementia and their family carer. The chapter also takes the view that people with dementia and their carers construct what situations constitute a risk and is accomplished through interactive and conversational processes that occur in meetings between people with dementia, family carers and the nurse. The last part of the chapter recognises the importance of good record keeping in dementia care nursing and outlines various ways in which it may occur.

References

Adams, T. (2001). The social construction of risk by community psychiatric nurses and family carers for people with dementia. *Health, Risk and Society* 3, 3, 307–319.

Adams, T. and Page, S. (2000). New pharmacological treatments for Alzheimer's disease: implications for dementia care nursing. *Journal of Advanced Nursing* 31, 5, 1183–1188.

Barker, P. (1997). *Assessment in Psychiatric and Mental Health Nursing: In Research of the Whole Person.* Cheltenham: Stanley Thornes.

Barker, P. (ed.) (2003). *Psychiatric and Mental Health Nursing: The Craft of Caring.* London: Arnold.

Barker, P. J., Reynolds, W. and Stevenson, C. (1997). The human science basis of psychiatric nursing theory and practice. *Journal of Advanced Nursing* 25, 4, 660–667.

Billig, M. (1987). *Arguing and Thinking: A Rhetorical Approach to Social Psychology.* Cambridge: Cambridge University Press.

Brayne, C. and Calloway, P. (1989). An epidemiological study of dementia in a rural population of elderly women. *British Journal of Psychiatry* 155, 214–219.

Clarke, C. L. (2000). Risk: Constructing care and care environments in dementia. *Health, Risk and Society* 2, 1, 83–93.

Clarke, C. and Heyman, B. (1999). Risk management for people with dementia. In B. Heyman (ed.) *Risk, Health and Healthcare: A Qualitative Approach.* London: Chapman and Hall, pp. 228–240.

Department of Health (2001). *The Single Assessment Process: Consultation Papers and Process.* London: The Stationery Office.

Department of Health (2005). *Everybody's Business. Integrated Mental Health Services for Older Adults. A Service Development Guide.* London: Care Services Improvement Partnership (CSIP).

Department of Health (2006). *Reviewing the Care Programme Approach: A Consultation Process.* London: The Stationery Office.

Feinberg, I. F. and Whitlatch, C. J. (2001). Are persons with cognitive impairment able to state consistent choices? *Gerontologist* 4, 1, 374–382.

Folstein, M. F., Folstein, S. E. and McHugh, P. R. (1975). Mini-mental state: a practical method for grading the cognitive state of patients for the clinician. *Journal of Psychiatric Research* 12, 189–198.

Keady, J. and Bender, M. P. (1998). Changing faces: the purpose and practice of assessing older adults with cognitive impairment. *Health Care in Later Life* 3, 2, 129–144.

Kitwood, T. (1997). *Dementia Reconsidered: The Person Comes First.* Buckingham: Open University Press.

Manthorpe, J. (2004). Risk Taking. In A. Innes, C. Archibald and C. Murphy (ed.) *Dementia and Social Inclusion.* London: Jessica Kingsley, pp. 137–149.

Marrelli, T. (2005). Dementia: Complex care needing ongoing assessment. *Geriatric Nursing* 26, 2, 81–82.

Morgan, S. and Wetherell, A. (2004). Assessing and managing risk. In I. Norman and I. Ryrie (eds) *The Art and Science of Mental Health Nursing: A Textbook of Principals and Practice,* pp. 208–204.

Moye, J., Karel, M. J., Azar, A. R. and Gurrera, R. J. (2004). Capacity to consent to treatment: empirical comparison of three instruments in older adults with and without dementia. *Gerontologist* 44, 2, 166–175.

Nichols, J., Phillips, M., Belisle, S., Sansone, P. and Scmitt, L. (1998). Determining the capacity of demented nursing home residents to name a health care proxy. *Clinical Gerontologist* 19, 35–50.

Robinson, B. (1983). Validation of a caregiver strain index. *Journal of Geronotology* 38, 344–348.

Ryrie, I. and Norman, I. (eds) (2004). *Assessment and Planning. The Art and Science of Mental Health Nursing: A Textbook of Principles and Practice,* pp. 183–287.

Sayers, J. (2005). Older people and mental health problems. In R. Tummey (ed.) *Planning Care in Mental Health Nursing.* Basingstoke: Palgrave, pp. 185–204.

Scottish Executive (2006). *Rights, Relationships and Recovery.* Edinburgh: Scottish Executive.

Taylor, C. and White, C. (2000). *Practising Reflexivity in Health and Welfare: Making Knowledge.* Buckingham: Open University Press.

Chapter 8

Communication between people with dementia, family members and nurses

Trevor Adams

Learning Outcomes

After reading the chapter you will be able to

- understand the contribution of biomedical and social/psychological phenomena within communication within dementia care nursing;
- discuss how various ideas drawn from ethnomethodology, conversation analysis and discourse analysis may contribute to understanding communication within dementia care nursing;
- describe how nurses may promote good communication between people with dementia and their family members;
- describe how people with dementia may find themselves disempowered and marginalised by communication processes within dementia care settings and how this may be addressed.

Introduction

In previous chapters we have argued that nursing people with dementia is a practical activity and that it is something that nurses say and do which enhances the physical, emotional and social well-being of people with dementia and their family members. It is clear, therefore, that one of the most important aspects of dementia care is communication (Haak, 2006). Various approaches have developed that describe how people interact with one another in dementia care settings. While these approaches are useful, many are too narrow and only highlight the transfer of information. We would, however, draw on a broader understanding of communication that not only sees communication as a way in which information is transferred between people but also that it gives rise to how dementia care settings are shaped or rather 'socially constructed'. As an alternative, this chapter draws on various schools within the social sciences, such as Conversation Analysis (CA) and discourse analysis that offer insights about how verbal and non-verbal language gives rise to how people see and feel about themselves, how different people are viewed and how dementia care is organised within society and local groups.

Communication Difficulties in People with Dementia

There are various reasons why people with dementia may find communication difficult. While sometimes poor communication may be due to the dementia itself, it may also be due to consequences of ageing, such as the loss of hearing or eyesight. Moreover, many people with dementia have diseases and pathological changes such as congestive cardiac failure or a cancer that may affect their ability to communicate effectively with other people. Of particular significance are neuro-psychological changes that give rise to neurological difficulties (see Insert 8:1).

Insert 8:1: Communication difficulties that may arise in people with dementia

Agnosia: failure to recognise familiar objects.

Apathy: lack of interest in everyday activities.

Aphasia: loss of ability to express or understand language or problems with communication.

Changing sets: difficulty changing from one movement or task to another.

Disorientation: the failure to know where one is, and/or date or time of day.

Impulse control: the ability to control, divert or postpone the expression of feelings such as anger, frustration, fear and anxiety.

Insight: the ability of the brain to monitor what is going on.

Judgement: the ability to make critical distinctions and to arrive at sensible decisions.

Insert 8:1 cont'd

Memory: various difficulties in memory may occur such as: 'recall' which is the ability to remember something that happened or something the other person was told a few minutes earlier; short-term memory loss which is memory for events that happened not along ago; and, long-term memory which is memory of things that happened a few weeks or years previously.

Mood: irritability, depression, restlessness and other changes in mood.

Perseveration: the tendency to 'get stuck' doing the same activity motion over and over again.

Spatial perceptions: difficulty perceiving where things are in relationship to oneself and other objects.

Taken from Mace (2005)

Communicating with a Person Who Has Dementia

People who are confused find it difficult to understand what people are saying or to put their views forward. This can be very frustrating for both the person with dementia and their carer. Numerous writers have suggested various ways in which people might better communicate with people who have dementia (see Rabins et al., 2006) (see Insert 8:2).

Insert 8:2 Tips in helping the development of good communication in dementia care nursing

1. Saying who you talking to!

Use the person's name to get their attention.
Make good eye contact and talk to the person directly.

2. Use appropriate and gentle gestures

Try gently touching the person on the arm and help them focus on the conversation.

3. Use short, simple sentences

Keep sentences short and easy to understand.
Speak clearly and slowly.

4. Repeat sentences

If the person does not seem to understand a particular word, try using another word that will convey the same meaning.

Insert 8:2 cont'd

5. Be specific

Say 'Here is your porridge' instead of 'It's time for breakfast.'
Try 'Do you want your glasses?' instead of 'Do you want these?'
Erase the phrase, 'Don't you remember?'

6. Offer simple choices

Ask questions that require a 'yes' or 'no' answer.
Limit the number of choices in a question: 'Would you like a cup of tea?' instead of 'Would you like something to drink?'
When giving instructions, give them one step at a time.

7. Use labels

Label frequently used items with a picture for example, a toilet on the bathroom door or cups on a cupboard door.

8. Use signals other than words

Wave or gently touch a person's arm to say hello.
Smile and nod to show you understand what he is saying.
Motion with your hand to invite him to join in an activity.
Show the person what you are talking about. For example, point to a glass when asking if he wants a glass of water.
Use touch when the person is upset.
Watch and listen for clues in behaviour. Wandering can often mean the person needs to use the toilet.
Be aware of your body language – facial expression, tone of voice and posture. The person may not understand the content of what you are saying but he will understand your non-verbal signals.

9. Try to determine what is really being said

Stop talking and listen to what the person is saying.
Repeat what you hear 'You're hungry now, aren't you?'
Think about what the person really means; 'I want to go home' may mean 'I'm anxious and need reassurance.'
Recognise the tone as well as the words.
Give the person time to answer.
Offer support even when you do not understand him.

10. Reduce distractions

Communicate in a calm, quiet environment where the person will not be distracted by other activities.
Encourage the person to wear his glasses and hearing aid.
Converse at face level. Approach from the front; do not surprise from behind.

Approaches towards Communication within Dementia Care Nursing

Underlying the approach taken in Insert 8:2 is the channelling model of communication (Thwaites et al., 2002). This approach highlights the passage (or channelling) of signals or messages from one person to another. While this approach offers helpful guidelines for dementia care nurses, it tends to be superficial. This is because it does not recognise that the message might change as it passes from the sender to the receiver and back again. The problems associated with the channelling model of communication were acknowledged by Kitwood who asserted that communication 'is not a matter of simply responding to signals' (Kitwood, 1997: p. 87) but rather based on 'interpretation and reflection' (p. 88) and was concerned with 'grasping the meanings conveyed by others' (Kitwood, 1997: p. 87). Thus for Kitwood, communication is much more than the mere transfer of messages but rather is concerned with how people with dementia interpret messages and thereby changes the initial message sent out by the receiver. In this way, Kitwood draws on an interpretative approach within the social sciences, most notably, symbolic interactionism (Blumer, 1969).

The approach developed in this chapter accepts Kitwood's rejection of the channelling approach, but rather than adopting an interpretative understanding of communication, draws on a social constructionist approach (Kitwood, 1997: pp. 87–89). We would therefore, want to develop a view of communication within dementia care settings that sees it not only as more than the passive transfer of information but also as actively participating in the organisation of dementia care settings.

Underpinning this approach is the work of numerous writers and philosophers, most notably the twentieth-century philosopher Wittgenstein (1958). Wittgenstein argued that language is not simply a mirror that reflects what the world is like but rather is itself an action that constructs and organises the world. His work has immense implications for dementia care nursing. Snyder (2006), for example, draws upon Wittgenstein and notes that 'interpersonal communication is a mutual, co-constructed process in which each person offers definitions of self and of what is real for others to interpret, affirm, or challenge' (p. 259). Snyder (2006) adds that people's understanding of what it is like to have Alzheimer's disease is mediated through language and that '[P]eople learn what it is to be an "Alzheimer's patient" based on messages used to convey or conceal the diagnosis, the medical ascription of neurological, cognitive, and functional deficits and the manner in which families and society interact within them' (p. 268). It is this wider understanding of communication that we would like to develop within dementia care nursing.

Drawing on ideas developed previously in this book, we would also want to argue that first, communication is reciprocal and gives rise not only to the subjective experience of the person with dementia but also to that of family member(s), nurses and other health and social care workers(s). In this way, everyone working alongside people with dementia is seen as possessing personhood which part at least, arises from what other people say and do. Second, it is not just people's sense of self that arises through communication but also their position within society and social groups such as within families and case conferences. It is through language and other social forms of interaction, therefore, that people's identity is carved out and the way they see themselves and are seen by others is constructed.

Last, we would affirm the contribution of the body within interpersonal communication and the way people see themselves and others within dementia care settings. The body contributes towards communication; for example, different parts of the body are used in talking and hearing, such as people's mouth, ears, hands and brain, and also the position and movement of the body in relationship to the listener is important. Also, what is done to the body, particularly when it is treated without dignity and in the absence of privacy, will affect a person's sense of self. This is of particular relevance to dementia care nurses who often find themselves undertaking intimate tasks that may undermine a person's dignity and affect their subjectivity and sense of well-being.

Developing Good Communication within Dementia Care Settings

Existing research studies and theoretical work offer few coherent views about how communication occurs between different people, agencies and systems associated with the provision of dementia care. While person-centred care focuses on how other people's talk gives rise to the subjectivity of people with dementia and relationship-centred care extends this idea by including the reciprocal interaction offered by family carer(s) and paid-for carer(s), each of these two approaches fail to explain how communication occurs between different systems within dementia care nursing.

More recently, various writers have developed a more robust way of understanding what happens when communication occurs in dementia care settings. Rather than using interpretative methods based on symbolic interactionism, writers have focused on language and have highlighted how verbal and non verbal language constructs the way the social world is organised. The importance of these approaches has been noted by Downs et al. (2006: p. 368) who suggest that they 'could be used as the basis for ensuring a patient and family-focused service and to refine advice to carers and people with dementia on effective service use'.

Communication in dementia care nursing occurs in various ways such as through verbal interaction, for example, between a nurse and a person with dementia and through bodily actions, such as facial gestures and seating positions. But communication may also occur through visual images, written notes and reports, governmental reports and communication on Internet blog sites and discussion groups. All these ways of communication contribute to how dementia care nursing is undertaken, and any theory about communication in dementia care nursing must be wide enough to take these approaches into account.

To address this issue, we would want to develop an approach which helps nurses understand what happens when people communicate with each other in dementia care settings. The approach I would like to draw upon is Discursive Psychology that has been developed by various writers such as Wetherell and Potter (1986), Potter (1996) and Edwards (1997) and has been applied more specifically to health and social care settings by Taylor and White (2000). This approach draws on different schools of thought within the social sciences that recognise the importance of language and shares with Wittgenstein the view that language does not merely describe objects and events but rather structures, constructs and gives them order.

Discursive Psychology and Its Understanding of Communication

Discursive Psychology mainly draws on endomethodology, conversation analysis and discourse analysis. Ethnomethodology is a branch of sociology that was initially developed by Garfinkel (1967). Its main concern is how people make sense of and reproduce social practices and focuses on what people do and why they do it. This focus on 'doing' is a theme developed in this book in relationship to dementia care nursing as it highlights what nurses actually say and do. Within ethnomethodology, making sense of the world is seen as something that is jointly accomplished by groups of people and communities, such as a person with dementia and their carer or different members of the family and a nurse. This approach challenges cognitive approaches towards nursing (see Crow et al., 1996) that argue that the views, opinions and decisions of nurses arise out of cognitive processes alone rather than seeing them, in part at least, arising out of a social process.

Potter (1996) identifies three ideas within ethnomethodology that are applicable to dementia care nursing as they are to other areas of social life. The first is 'indexicality'. This is the idea that the meaning of an utterance is dependent upon its context. Thus, the meaning of a particular word arises not because of its dictionary definition but because of how it is used within an utterance. For example, if a nurse describes an older person as being just like a 'baby', they are not using the dictionary definition of 'baby' but rather they are drawing on culturally understood ideas of what it means to be a baby and allowing that person to be seen by others as 'babyish'. The second is 'reflexivity' which refers to the idea that utterances do not merely describe the external world but rather construct it. Thus representing someone as 'the carer' will allow them to be seen, feel and become 'the carer' within a particular social group. Last, Garfinkel (1967) outlines 'the documentary method of interpretation' that describes how people's views develop against a background of their expectancies, models and ideas. Thus when undertaking an assessment, a nurse will develop ideas about what is happening in a particular situation by drawing on different accounts and stories that are available in the clinical setting. In these ways, endomethodology provides worthwhile insights about how communication occurs in practice settings.

The second approach that Discursive Psychology draws upon is Conversation Analysis. This approach developed out of ethnomethodology and is concerned with how sets of meaning arise within the sequential features of talk, such as the turns that people take, the pauses in the talk, the way issues are introduced (Hutchby and Wooffitt, 1998). CA has been used to understand what happens in communication and to describe how meaning is produced in a variety of social settings, such as nursing. Examples of the use of CA within dementia care may be found in the work of Shakespeare (1998), Clare and Shakespeare (2004) and more specifically within dementia care nursing by Adams (2000, 2001a, b).

Sacks, who with Schegloff and Jefferson initially developed CA, argued that conversations are systematically organised and sequentially ordered (Sacks, 1992). He identified three underlying characteristics of conversations. First, utterances within conversations may be viewed as resources that speakers use to make particular social accomplishments. For example, if a relative tells a nurse that her mother does not understand what she is saying, she may not just be telling the nurse something which should be taken at face value but may also allow the nurse to infer that the woman's mother is quite dependent.

Second, utterances that occur within conversations in dementia care nursing are not accidental or haphazard but rather have a specific purpose within the conversational exchange. Adams (2000) describes the interaction that arises when a carer is making a criticism about an aspect of care his wife is receiving and shows how the carer skilfully uses what he is saying so that he is not seen as someone who is ungrateful as this would undermine his identity as a good carer.

Third, interaction between people is itself the object of analysis. The implication is that through its analysis, insights into the decision-making processes between different participants may be gained. Thus within dementia care nursing, the interest of CA is not on ideas and theories that lie outside practice itself or the agendas or intentions that lie within the speaker but rather the way different meanings that are made available through the organisation of talk within practice settings.

Various patterns of communication have been identified within CA that reveal how participants allow other people to infer and thus hear various sets of meaning in conversations (Potter, 1996). The patterns have been applied to different health and social care settings by writers such as Taylor and White (2000). Each of these patterns frequently occurs in dementia care nursing.

Dilemma of Stake

Dilemmas of stake occur when people describe events in which they have an interest (Edwards and Potter, 1993). The idea is helpful in dementia care nursing as it reminds nurses that each participant – person with dementia, family member and nurse – have their own agenda, and that through their interaction with others they are able (if they are allowed by the other participants!) to hear sets of meaning that support their overall agenda. While the agenda of some family carers may be the same as that of their relative with dementia, some relatives may have a very different agenda. In these cases, there may be a dilemma of stake.

The notion of 'dilemma of stake' is applicable to communication that occurs in dementia care nursing and reveals how versions of events are 'worked up' in a way that support the participant's agenda. This feature within conversations is called an 'epistemological orientation' and describes how verbal utterances make what is being said more believable. However, the interest of CA is the utterance and what it accomplishes within social groups. CA does not make any claim about people's inner thoughts and agendas, though they might exist, but just what it does.

Detail and Narrative

Potter (1996) identifies adding detail as a further way of strengthening the believability of an account or story. He argues that adding detail allows listeners to think that because they can recall so much detail they must know what they are talking about and that the account is factual. For example, a husband might be telling a nurse about an incident that has occurred with his wife who has dementia. The more detail he is able to insert into the account, more it looks as though he knows what he is talking about and that his account is accurate.

Extreme Case Formulations

Another strategy that strengthens the believability of a story are extreme case formulations (Pomerantz, 1986). These occur when an object or event is referred to in a way that invokes its maximal or minimal properties. Thus, a man may tell a nurse that his wife has 'not slept for a whole week' when what really happened was that she has slept, but a lot less than she usually does. The statement is not factual but rather allows the nurse to infer that the woman has not slept very much at all.

Active Voicing

Wooffitt (1992) describes how reported speech may be used to strengthen the factual status of accounts and stories. He describes how speakers use 'active voicing' by allowing what is being said to be heard *as if* it is being said as if it had happened. Thus, a woman may be talking about her difficulties caring for her husband and inserts into her account a piece of reported speech. For example, she may say, 'He said, "I am never going to that Day Hospital again".' Through the use of active voicing, the nurse hears what was being said as if it were being said at that particular time and thus makes the account more believable.

Category Management

Sacks (1992) identifies the importance of how things are categorised in conversations. In a classic discussion on category management, Sacks examines the following sentences: 'The baby cried. The mommy picked it up.' Sacks argued that listeners will frequently assume that the 'mommy' is the mommy of the baby that cried. But this might not be the case, as 'the mommy' could be some other baby's mommy! The implication is that by categorising someone as 'mommy' the speaker allows the listener to make various inferences about the 'mommy', notably that she is the mommy of the baby that cried. But this might not be the case and is only the *preferred* understanding because of the way categories were managed within conversations. Conversation analytic studies have shown the ability of categories to offer a range of inferences within conversations, including those occurring in dementia care (Adams, 2000, 2001a, b). For example, a nurse may be talking to another health care worker about a man who is caring for a woman with dementia. The nurse has a choice of referring to the man in a number of various ways. But by using the term 'husband', the nurse allows the other care worker to make various inferences about the man's obligations and responsibility towards the woman.

To summarise, CA offers nurses a detailed and comprehensive approach towards understanding how people in dementia care settings communicate with each other. CA shows how different patterns of communication lead to accounts of events being accepted and offers people different identities.

The third approach within Discursive Psychology draws upon discourse analysis. While ethnomethodology and conversation analysis focus on how people make sense of conversations, discourse analysis highlights how different forms of language such as body language, the written word and the visual image set up a particular way of viewing situations. Underpinning discourse analysis is the view that language does not have a fixed meaning but rather is fluid and always changing. This may be seen in dementia care nursing in the way the meaning of terms like 'dementia' and 'Alzheimer's disease are nowadays used. A key idea here is 'discourse' which Parker (1992, p. 5) understands as 'a system of statements which construct an object' and Burr (1995, p. 48) says 'a set of meanings, metaphors, representations, images, stories, statements and so on'. The importance of discourse is that they construct the world and says 'practices which form the objects of which they speak' (Foucault, 1972, p. 49).

Discourse analysis is concerned with examining how different discourses construct the way people see and feel about themselves, how different people are viewed and how society and local social groups are organised. For example, discourse analysis is concerned with how in dementia care nursing, medical discourse through words such as 'dementia' and 'Alzheimer's disease', metaphors such as people with dementia being part of 'a rising tide' of old people that will swamp the rest of society, and images such as those that appear on adverts selling anti-dementia drugs such as Aricept construct dementia care settings in a particular way. However, discourse analysis does not merely identify various discourses that are located within particular social settings, it also links them to wider structures and practices in society and argues that 'it is in the interest of relatively powerful groups that some discourses and not others receive the stamp of "truth" ' (Burr, 1995, p. 55). Thus, discourse analysis offers insights about how certain groups of people such as government agencies construct and organise society and provides insights about how power is distributed within society and social groups. This is clearly seen in the work of Harding and Palfrey (1998), who reveal how dementia 'is an example of a socially constructed disease, and that the major players in such a construction – its architects as it were – are the medical profession' (p. 4) and shows how medical discourse provides a means by which society is socially controlled and organised. A similar understanding is offered by Gilleard and Higgs (2000). Moreover at a local level also, within meetings between dementia care nurses and families, discourses may be located which make particular outcomes seem more appropriate than others and, therefore, construct the decisions that are taken. For example the presence of discourses that highlight the family may bring to the foreground the stress experienced by the family, and may make respite care seem the most suitable way of dealing with a particular clinical situation.

It should be noted that discourses located in particular situations will raise the visibility and importance of some features of the situation and people within it, and minimise others. For example, a family member might describe a situation using 'family discourse' that highlights the role of the family in the provision of care, whereas a medical practitioner might use 'medical discourse' that highlights biomedical aspects of the situation and the need for medical and perhaps, hospital attention. In addition, certain discourses may also construct particular people as powerful, while others are marginalised and disempowered. For example, dementia care settings which contain medical discourse highlights the inability of the person with dementia to make their own decisions, whereas settings that contain disability discourse would highlight the obstacles society puts in the way of people who are chronically confused people. In this way, discourse is seen to offer different people 'subject positions' which may either empower or disempower them in social settings (Harré and van Langenhove, 1999). The idea here is that the utterances, words, stories and discourse that offer people different ways of seeing themselves and being seen by others that allows them to occupy different roles and identities and having various rights, duties, entitlements and obligations. Sabat (2006) describes how positioning has been found to be an important way by which identity is managed within dementia care settings (Sabat, 2001; see also Adams, 2000, 2001a).

To summarise, discourse analysis provides insights about how different discourses contained in what people do and say contribute to the social construction of dementia care settings and offer people with a way of seeing and feeling about themselves and is a means by which dementia care settings and the provision of dementia care is ordered. We would argue that this approach allows dementia care nurses to develop insights about dementia care settings that allow them to recognise how people with dementia care settings may find themselves marginalised and disempowered and enable them to develop strategies that promote their inclusion within the decision-making process.

Conversational Patterns That Occur between Participants within Dementia Care Nursing

A frequent form of interaction within dementia care nursing occurs between 'dementia care triads' comprising the person with dementia, their family carer and the nurse. Adams and Gardiner (2005) identify two broad types of interaction that occur with triadic interaction in dementia care nursing. The first type 'disabling dementia communication' occurs in practice settings in which the nurse or family member either prevents usually, the person with dementia, from expressing their thoughts and opinions or represents them as being unable to make their own decisions. The second form of interaction comprises 'disabling dementia communication' which occurs when, usually the person with dementia, are offered an identity which allows their empowerment and enables their views to be heard.

Disabling Dementia Communication

The idea of 'disabling dementia communication' is conceptually similar though different from Kitwood's (1997) idea of 'malignant social psychology' and Sabat's 'malignant positioning' (Sabat, 2001). The main difference between these ideas is that disabling dementia communication is associated with the interaction between three people (see Insert 8:3).

Different types of disabling dementia communication are outlined in Insert 8:3:

Insert 8:3 Different types of disabling dementia communication (taken from Adams and Gardiner, 2005)

- *Interrupting*: This occurs when a nurse or family member interrupts a person with dementia while they are expressing their views.
- *Speaking on behalf of*: This occurs when a nurse or family member talks about a person with dementia having views and opinions that they have not expressed themselves.
- *Reinterpreting*: This occurs when a nurse or family member rephrases or changes the meaning of something the person with dementia has said.
- *Using too technical or complex language*: This occurs when a nurse or family member uses words and phrases the person with dementia finds difficult to understand.

Different types of enabling dementia communication are outlined in Insert 8:4.

Summary

This chapter has developed a theory about how people within dementia care nursing communicate with each other. This theory argues that communication is not merely the passive transfer of information between the sender and receiver but rather actively constructs the social world. Thus, verbal and non-verbal language within dementia care settings are not so much concerned with sharing truths but rather constructing and establishing truths. The chapter draws on Discourse Psychology mainly through the use of ethnomethodology, conversation analysis and discourse analysis to provide a theoretical underpinning for this approach and describes how these approaches offer insights about what happens within communication in dementia care nursing. Underpinning the chapter is the view that communication is both a bodily and social process that allows people to make inferences about what is happening in dementia care settings and that communication occurs between people within different social systems.

References

Adams, T. (2000). The social construction of identity by community psychiatric nurses and family members caring for people with dementia. *Journal of Advanced Nursing* 32, 4, 791–798.

Adams, T. (2001a). The construction of moral identity within accounts of informal carers for people with dementia. *Education and Ageing* 16, 39–54.

Adams, T. (2001b). The conversational and discursive construction of community psychiatric nursing for chronically confused people and their families. *Nursing Inquiry* 8, 98–107.

Adams, T. and Gardiner, P. (2005). Communication and interaction within dementia care triads: developing a theory for relationship-centred care. *Dementia: The International Journal of Social Research and Practice* 4, 2, 185–205.

Blumer, H. (1969). *Symbolic Interactionism: Perspective and Method.* London: University of California Press.

Burr, V. (1995). *An Introduction to Social Constructionism.* London: Routledge.

Clare, L. and Shakespeare, P. (2004). Negotiating the impact of forgetting. *Dementia* 3, 1, 211–251.

Crow, R., Chase, J. and Lamond, D. (1996). The cognitive component of nursing assessment an analysis. *Journal of Advanced Nursing* 8, 2, 107–110.

Downs, M., Clare, L. and Mackenzie, J. (2006). Understandings of dementia: explanatory models and their implications for the person with dementia and therapeutic effort. In J. C. Hughes, S. J. Louw and S. R. Sabat (eds) *Dementia: Mind, Meaning, and the Person.* Oxford: Oxford University Press, pp. 235–258.

Edwards, D. (1997). *Discourse and Cognition.* London: Sage.

Edwards, D. and Potter, J. (1993). Language and causation: A discursive action model of description and attribution. *Psychological Review* 100, 230–41.

Garfinkel, H. (1967). *Studies in Ethnomethodology*. Englewood Cliffs, N.J.: Prentice-Hall.

Gilleard, C. and Higgs, P. (2000). *Cultures of Ageing: Self, Citizen and the Body. Harlow: Prentice Hall.*

Goldsmith, M. (1996). *Hearing the Voice of People with Dementia*. London: Jessica Kingsley.

Haak, N. J. (2006). Communication – The heart of caregiving. *Alzheimer's Care Quarterly* 7, 2, 77–83.

Harding, N. and Palfrey, C. (1997). *The Social Construction of Dementia: Confused Professionals.* London: Jessica Kingsley.

Harré, R. and van Langenhove, L. (1999). Introduction to positioning theory. In R. Harré and L. van Langenhove (eds) *Positioning Theory*. Oxford: Blackwell, pp. 14–31.

Hutchby, I. and Wooffitt, R. (1998). *Conversation Analysis: Principles, Practices and Applications.* Oxford: Polity Press.

Kitwood, T. (1997). *Dementia Reconsidered: The Person Comes First*. Buckingham: Open University Press.

Mace, N. L. (2005). *Teaching Dementia Care*. Baltimore: Johns Hopkins University Press.

Parker, I. (1992). *Discourse Dynamics*. London: Routlegde.

Pomerantz, A. (1986). Extreme case formulations. *Human Studies* 9, 219–230.

Potter, J. (1996). *Representing Reality: Discourse Rhetoric and Social Constructionism*. London: Sage.

Potter, J. and Wetherell, M. (1986). *Discourse and Social Psychology: Beyond Attitudes and Behaviour.* London: Sage.

Rabins, P. V., Lyketos, C. and Steel, S. D. (2006). *Practical Dementia Care*. (2nd ed.). New York: Oxford University Press.

Sabat, S. (2001). *The Experience of Alzheimer's Disease – Life through a Tangled Veil* Oxford: Blackwell.

Sabat, S. (2006). The self in dementia. In M. L. Johnson (ed.) *The Cambridge Handbook of Ageing*, pp. 332–337.

Foucault, M. (1992). *The Archerology of Knowledge*. London: Tavistock.

Sacks, H. (1992). *Lectures on Conversation*. Volume 1 and 2, ed. G. Jefferson, Oxford: Basil Blackwell.

Shakespeare, P. (1998). *Aspects of Confused Speech*. New Jersey: Erlbaum.

Snyder, L. (2006). Personhood and interpersonal communication in dementia. In J. C. Hughes, S. J. Louw and S. R. Sabat (eds) *Dementia: Mind, Meaning and the Person*. Oxford: Oxford University Press. pp. 259–276.

Taylor, C. and White, S. (2000). *Practising Reflexivity in Health and Welfare: Making Knowledge*. Buckingham: Open University Press.

Thwaites, T., Davis, L. and Mules, W. (2002). *Introducing Cultural and Media Studies*. Palgrave: London.

Weedon, C. (1993). *Feminist Practice and Post Structuralist Theory*. Oxford: Blackwell Publications.

Wittgenstein, L. (1958). *Philosophical Investigations*. Oxford: Blackwell.

Wooffitt, R. (1992). *Telling Tales of the Unexpected: The Organisation of Factual Discourse*. Hemel Hempstead: Harvester Wheatsheaf.

Chapter 9

Activities and interventions with people who have dementia and their families

Trevor Adams

Learning Outcomes

After reading the chapter you will be able to

- differentiate individual and family work within dementia care nursing;
- critically review various theoretical approaches towards activity in older people, including people with dementia;
- discuss the use of various therapeutic approaches with people who have dementia;
- describe how nurses can work with families in dementia care situations;
- describe the use of various approaches, such as information-giving, crisis intervention and problem-solving as a means of promoting well-being;
- discuss the management of medication within dementia care settings.

Introduction

This chapter outlines different activities and interventions that dementia care nurses may use to promote well-being in people with dementia and their family members. While people with dementia receive nursing care in different settings, there are two main modes in which it occurs. The first mode is individual work that may occur with either the person with dementia or an informal carer. The second mode is family work that may occur with different family members, including the person with dementia, and is concerned with interventions that promote the well-being of different members of the family. While it may often be appropriate in family work for nurses to work with just the family carer(s), the option to include the person with dementia should always be considered, and if following an invitation, the person with dementia does not attend, they should certainly be present at the meeting 'in spirit'.

Individual Work with People with Dementia

In the 1960s, Cumming and Henry (1961) developed an approach towards older people called 'disengagement theory' (Cumming and Henry, 1961). This approach viewed ageing as a gradual, though inevitable withdrawal or disengagement from interaction with other people. The approach argued that disengagement was beneficial not only for older people but also for the rest of society. Underlying disengagement theory is the idea that there is a transition of power from the young to the old that results in normalising the marginalisation and removal of older people from society (Victor, 2005). This approach raises difficulties because it legitimates the marginalisation and disempowerment of older people, and fails to promote their well-being.

We would, however, draw upon an alternative approach towards older people, that of Activity Theory (Havighurst, 1963). Underlying Activity Theory is the view that normal and successful ageing is concerned with preserving, for as long as possible, the attitudes and patterns of activity of middle age. Activity Theory rejects the separation between society and older people and supports the value of purposeful activity as a means of securing their social inclusion. Within Activity Theory, well-being is positively related to social integration and participation within social networks. In this context, older people are seen to lose their place/position/role in society through experiences such as retirement and widowhood and need to be compensated for this. Moreover, this approach fits in well with the work of Archer (2000) particularly the idea of the 'primacy of practice' and also the notion of 'embodied selfhood' developed in the work of Kontos (2006) (see Chapter 3).

Before we examine different activities that nurses can undertake with people who have dementia and their family, we would want to outline the basic ideas that underpin therapeutic engagement between the nurse, the person with dementia and their family members. Carl Rogers' (1983) client-centred approach towards the development and sustainability of therapeutic relationships identifies three ideas that are just as applicable to dementia care nursing as they are to other areas of mental health care (Insert 9:1).

Activities for People With Dementia

Different approaches supported by psychological theory may be used to underpin nursing practice with people who have dementia and their family. One early approach was Reality Orientation (see Holden and Woods, 1995), which put forward various behavioural and cognitive techniques to help orientate people with dementia.

Reality Orientation

Reality Orientation (RO) was developed in the late 1950s in the United States by Folsom and is still one of the most widely used approaches for people with dementia. RO has two forms: the first form is '24 hour RO' or 'informal RO'. This form of RO comprises staff providing the person with dementia current information as they interact with them; reminding them of the time, place and person; providing them with a commentary of events; and responding positively to their requests for information. The second form of RO is 'classroom RO' or 'formal RO'. In this form, daily sessions lasting about 30–45 minutes are held for people with dementia. The content of the session is dependent on the ability of group members.

In a group, participants will be concerned with presenting and repeating current information such as the date, the weather and the names of other group members. In typical group sessions, sensory stimulation is used and discussion is encouraged as a means of building interpersonal relationships within the group. In more advanced groups, less emphasis is placed on presentation and repetition, and interaction within the group is similar to that of everyday communication.

One of the main difficulties with RO is that it is easy for nurses to become tired and discouraged by its intensive nature. In this respect, 24 hour RO is considered to be 'the more practical' (Ballard et al., 2001: p. 129) of the two forms of RO. There has been considerable discussion about the efficacy of RO, two findings repeatedly emerge. The first is that RO can increase a person's verbal orientation and the second is that 'real life' changes following RO are difficult to obtain, although behavioural changes can be achieved when specific targeting occurs. In addition, it has been suggested that RO is far too mechanical and can be too confrontational ('To-day is *Monday*!!'). Also RO may simply remind people with dementia that they are forgetful and confused. This may account for the finding of Baines et al. (1987) that people attending RO sessions are more likely to experience an initial lowering of mood.

Reminiscence

Erikson et al. (1986) argue that reminiscence makes a positive contribution to the mental health of older people. They argue that reminiscence is an important activity in older people and is something they must do to maintain optimal mental health. They adds that reminiscence allows older people to develop a 'sense of oneself across the life-cycle and involves a coming to terms with perceived mistakes, failures and omissions – with chances missed and opportunities not taken' (Erikson et al., 1986: p. 141).

Reminiscence, therefore, may be seen as a way of helping older people, including people with dementia think about and relive past experiences, especially those that have a personal significance (Ballard et al., 2001). Osborn (1993), for example, describes 18 different group activities that promote reminiscence in people with dementia. These activities include 'asking the group things about the past'; 'making displays about the past'; 'dramas about past events'; 'painting and writing stories about the past'; 'handling old objects'; examining 'maps of places that have past significance for people'; and 'comparing things from the past with how things are now'.

Validation Therapy

Validation Therapy has been advocated as a means of helping people with dementia and was developed by Naomi Feil (1982, 1992). The approach identifies that people with cognitive impairment experience one of four stages: Mal orientation; Time Confusion; Repetitive Motion; and Vegetation. Validation Therapy challenges behavioural and cognitive approaches that merely remind people with dementia of what is happening and affirms that people's feelings also need validation.

Validation Therapy is based on the idea that each person is unique and valuable and should be treated non-judgmentally and as an individual. The behaviour of people with dementia is understood holistically as the result of physical, social and psychological changes that have taken place over the lifespan. Feil draws on the work of Erikson (1986) and argues that people need to complete certain tasks during different periods of their life and that failure to do so may lead a person to have psychological problems. When more recent memory failure occurs, Validation Therapy suggests that people should try to restore balance in their lives by retrieving earlier memories; for example, when they cannot *hear*, they *listen* to sounds from the past. Painful emotions expressed by people with dementia are acknowledged and validated by a trusted listener so that they will diminish, and through the use of empathy trust is built up and dignity restored. In this way, Validation Therapy may be seen as a way of promoting the well-being of people with dementia.

Validation Therapy identifies various techniques staff may use with people who have dementia (see Insert 9:2).

Insert 9:2 Validation techniques that can be used by nurses talking to people with dementia

Centring: Focusing on breathing before talking to people who are disorientated.

Using non-threatening, factual words to build trust: Using factual questions such as who, what, where, when, and how.

Rephrasing: Repeating the gist of what someone with dementia has said by using the same key words and tone of voice.

Insert 9:2 cont'd

Using polarity: Asking the person with dementia to think about the most extreme example of his or her complaint.

Imagining the opposite: Asking the person with dementia to imagine the opposite to allow them to recollect a familiar solution to a problem.

Reminiscing: Exploring the past can re-establish familiar coping methods that the disoriented person once used and can help people with dementia survive present day losses.

Maintaining genuine, close eye contact: Looking directly into the eyes of someone with dementia.

Using ambiguity: Time Confused people often use words that have no meaning to others. By using ambiguity, nurses can communicate with people who are Time Confused even when they do not understand what is being said.

Using a clear, low, loving tone of voice: This can be very reassuring to people who are confused.

Observing and matching the person's motion and emotions (Mirroring): Mimicking the physical movements of people with dementia as a means of promoting their understanding.

Linking the behaviour with the unmet human needs: Most people need to be loved and nurtured, to be active and engaged and to express their deep emotions to someone who listens with empathy.

Identifying and using the preferred sense: Communicating using a person's preferred sense – seeing, hearing, touching, smelling and tasting.

Using music: When words have gone, familiar, early learned melodies return.

Kitwood, and Positive Person Work and the Promotion of Well-being

Kitwood (1997) outlined various communication strategies that may be used with people who have dementia. Kitwood calls the use of these strategies 'positive person work' and describes how they may enhance the subjective well-being of people with dementia.

Kitwood (1997) describes various types of 'positive person work' (see Insert 9:3).

Insert 9:3 Different types of positive person work (taken from Kitwood, 1997)

Recognition: when a person with dementia is acknowledged as a person by such activities as the use of their preferred name, having their views affirmed and simply by being thanked.

Negotiation: when a person with dementia is asked about their wants and preferences rather than being told what other people want them to do. It is accomplished by nurses undertaking activities such as coming near to and looking at the person with dementia, asking them what they would like and listening to their response.

Collaboration: when the person with dementia and the carer share a task or activity. The key idea is that the carer's words and body movements should not allow the person with dementia to feel they are having something 'done to' them and offer instead a sense of dignity, value and well-being.

Play: when people with dementia enjoy themselves through activities that engender spontaneity, self-expression and fun.

Timalation: when people receive pleasure directly from their senses in activities that are provided by an informal or paid-for carer. Timalation may occur through any of the senses and allows carers to undertake practices that promote a sense of well-being in the person with dementia. Snoezelen is a common method of providing opportunities that allows the person with dementia to have a positive sense of self and well-being. In addition, various arts-based therapies such as dance therapy and art therapy allow people with dementia to express emotion through their body

Celebration: when the person with dementia is open to joy and thankful for the gift of life. Celebrations may include birthdays and anniversaries and should not just be restricted to their own but to those around them too. Celebrations promote the sense of well-being and dignity in people with dementia.

Relaxation: relaxation occurs when for a short time people stop active work. Relaxation allows people to have time out, refocus themselves, and thus enhance their sense of value and self.

Validation: when the carer goes beyond their own concerns and frame of reference and attends to the feelings and emotions of the person with dementia and allows them to feel that they are understood and valued.

Holding: when what the nurse says allows them to be fully present, steady, assured and responsive and able to tolerate resonances of all disturbing emotions. Holding offers people with dementia a sense of value and dignity.

Facilitation: Helping the person with dementia make their views and feelings known.

Killick and Allen, and Communication in People with Dementia

While Kitwood is a major influence on Killick and Allen (2001), Allen (2006) points out that Killick's work 'began independently' (p. 186) and was based on meeting and being with people who have dementia. Allen (2006) describes how Killick experienced dementia care through 'a personal immersion' (p. 187) by visiting care homes that allowed him to listen and attend to people with dementia and recognise they were communicating with him and each other.

Underpinning the work of Killick and Allen (2001) is the view that people with dementia use words to communicate what it is like to have dementia and that what they say frequently has a coherent and intrinsic meaning. Thus, they highlight the importance of actively listening to what the person with dementia is saying and understanding their experience. Killick and Allen (2001) identify various skills that help people with dementia communicate their experience of dementia (Insert 9:4).

Insert 9:4 Skills that promote communication with people who have dementia (adapted from Killick and Allen, 2001)

Stopping talking: this skill also involves demonstrating through our demeanour that we are actually listening to what they are saying. It requires concentrated and sensitive listening; it also requires periods of silence, often considerable silence, which goes against the cultural understanding that communication occurs through talk.

Non-verbal communication: body language is an important way a person with dementia and a nurse may communicate to each other. These forms of non-communication include eye contact, facial expression, voice, touch and posture.

Mirroring: involves focusing on the movements of people with dementia and reflecting back what they do and in the style they are doing it. Mirroring may include words but it is more powerful and moving when it is focussed on the person's body movements. To do mirroring effectively, it requires attention and sensitivity.

Pacing: involves altering the pace and rhythm of conversation.

Going with the flow: allowing the person with dementia control the topic of conversation.

Insert 9:4 cont'd

Incomplete utterances: helping the person with dementia who has lost their way in a conversation come to the end of what they are saying by adding a few words.

Communicating during other activities: talking to someone while they are doing an activity may help some people with dementia communicate.

Dealing with strong emotion: this occurs when a person with dementia feels they can trust you and expresses strong feelings.

Talking about yourself: revealing things about yourself that will develop trust and promote empathy.

More recently, Killick and Allen (2005, 2006) have developed an innovative approach to communicating with people who have severe dementia and applies techniques initially used with people who are in a coma. The approach uses attentive listening to hear what people with dementia are saying. Another approach that is being developed for use with people who have severe dementia is pre-therapy (Dodds 2007 a, b).

Art Therapy

Art therapy can provide people who have dementia with a source of meaningful stimulation and improve their ability to interact with other people. Activities such as drawing and painting may help people with dementia express themselves physically and emotionally. Art therapy may be used with people who have dementia as a means of providing recreation and enjoyment and to elicit therapeutic insights that may support the nursing care plan.

Art therapy is outlined by Queen-Daugherty (2001) and Kahn-Denis (2005), who describes how it may aid the diagnosis of dementia. Art therapy may draw on a variety of theoretical approaches. As Foth notes

> Art therapy practice is based on knowledge of human development and psychological theories which are implemented in the full spectrum of models of assessment and treatment including educational, psychodynamic, cognitive, transpersonal, and other therapeutic means of reconciling emotion conflicts, fostering self-awareness, developing social skill,

managing behavior, solving problems, reducing anxiety, aiding reality orientation, and increasing self-esteem. (Cited in Innes and Hatfield, 2001)

Art therapy not only helps the person with dementia but also contributes to the development of positive relationships with nurses and offers them an opportunity to get to know their clients. In this way, Art Therapy may be seen as a means of promoting well-being.

Music Therapy

Two approaches have been adopted towards music therapy. The first is concerned with music as a therapy in itself, and the second is concerned with the use of music within therapy. Ballard et al. (2001), in a review of empirical studies examining the effectiveness of music therapy, identify its beneficial effects to people with dementia, particularly in relationship to the relief of stress, promotion of relaxation, reduction of physiological arousal and the facilitation of verbal communication.

Various writers have described the beneficial effect of carers singing to people with dementia. Clair (2000) comments, '[s]inging is integral to the life of those who are in progressive dementia and their caregivers' and argues that caregiver singing provides 'islands of arousal, awareness, familiarity, comfort, community and success' (p. 93). Brown et al. (2001) describe an evaluation of the effectiveness of 'music-therapeutic caregiving' on a 24-bed specialist dementia care unit which involved carers singing to people with dementia, such as while they were cleaning and dressing them and during medication and meal times. They found that 'caregiver singing during personal care had a paradoxical effect: despite a lack of verbal instruction people with dementia seemed to understand what was happening; there was a strong sense of cooperation, and more of the person's own personality emerged' (p. 34).

Dance Therapy

Coaten (2001) links therapeutic dance with reminiscence and suggests that memories are not only contained in people's cognition but are also laid down or stored in people's bodies. He argues that dance is one way of gaining access to people's stored memories. Rather than talking about re-enacting a past event or memory,

Coaten prefers to talk about 're-living it ... [the memory] in the present' (p. 20) so that '[T]he living symbol of the original event manifests in the moment. It is as if those associations are an enduring, living presence and they can be returned to at any one time' (p. 20). He suggests that dance and movement can make a real difference to people with dementia.

Nyström and Lauritzen (2005) in a study of video-data taken from group dance sessions with people who have dementia found that through their use of body movement, speech and singing, the body is used as a substitute or as a support to speech as well as to express thoughts, memories and emotions. In this way, dance may be seen as a means of allowing people with dementia find alternative means of expressing themselves.

Snoezelen

Over the past few years, many dementia care units have installed Snoezelen rooms, which offer different forms of multi-sensory stimulation directed towards the sense of sight, hearing, touch, taste and smell, through the use of lighting effects, tactile surfaces, meditative music and the aroma of relaxing essential oils (Pinkney, 1997). The central feature of a Snoezelen room is usually a fibre optic system containing flashing lights of different colours. In addition, sound may be incorporated into Snoezelen and often comprises soothing sounds, such as waves or a stream. It is argued that Snoezelen provides a sensory environment that places fewer demands on the intellectual abilities of people with dementia and is directed towards their residual sensorimotor abilities (Hope, 1997).

Few studies have evaluated the effectiveness of Snoezelen with people who have dementia. However, Ballard et al. (2001) argue that Snoezelen has good face validity and that anecdotal accounts have supported its effectiveness. Two studies (Holtkamp et al., 1997; Kragt et al., 1997) found that there was a significant improvement in well-being and a reduction in behavioural problems among people with severe dementia during the multi-sensory treatment periods. However, the use of Snoezelen differs between clinical settings and this makes the therapeutic value of Snoezelen difficult to gauge.

Family Work

In Chapter 5, we outlined studies that view the experience of family members caring for people with dementia in terms of progressive stress, loss and failure to adjust and cope with arising situations. Various models describing the emotional experience of family carers have been developed by Zarit et al. (1986) and Boss (2002). While we value these approaches, we are concerned that they just focus on recognising and addressing the needs of primary family carer. We would argue that, first, the person with dementia should be included when the term 'family' is used and that, second, the contribution of different family members, whether they are giving direct or indirect care, is fully recognised. We adopted this approach in Chapter 6 and described 'a whole systems approach' towards dementia care nursing. Developing interventions that focus on one 'carer' may prevent the person with dementia contributing to family decision making, and may minimise the contribution of other members of the family who are making an indirect contribution to the promotion of well-being.

Gamble and Brennan (2006) outline three levels of intervention that may occur between people with various forms of mental health condition, families and health and social care professionals.

- Level 1: engagement and communication support plus introduction to service provision and personnel.
- Level 2: communication support plus tailor-made information to maintain current coping strategies and develop relapse response.
- Level 3: full family intervention to enhance communication and coping styles.

Family work may be undertaken in various modes that comprise

- one or more family carers,
- the person with dementia and other family members,
- members of different families, for example, as in a relative support group.

Information Giving

Nurses are in an excellent position to provide information that will help the family, including the person with dementia and can help them understand what is going on, dispel existing myths and misunderstandings about dementia and promote well-being through the reduction of stress. This information may relate to such issues as the nature and progression of dementia, advice about medication and various agencies that might promote well-being. Information may be offered not only during conversations but also through written leaflets, books and perhaps even videos. The Alzheimer's Society web site in the United Kingdom (http://www.alzheimers. org.uk/) provides a considerable amount of useful and accessible information about all aspects of dementia. The Society also provides a free magazine for people with dementia. However, the provision of this information needs to go hand-in-hand with discussion about issues that may have arisen in which family members are given the time to talk freely about what is happening to them. Carers should not be subjected to patronising talk from nurses who do not respect that the person with dementia and their family members have an intrinsic value and are a unique source of knowledge. A particularly important time when information may be shared with family carers is when the diagnosis is made. This is a difficult time for all the family and it is important that the person with dementia should, if possible, be offered information about the diagnosis and treatment.

Support

As we saw in Chapter 5, looking after someone with dementia can be emotionally tiring and many relatives need help and support to deal with day-to-day issues that occur in the provision of care. Underpinning the one-to-one interaction that nurses offer people with dementia and their families are the three Rogerian principles of therapeutic engagement: empathetic understanding, genuineness and unconditional positive regard.

Problem Solving

All families have different ways of coping with situations and nurses must always assume that families have strengths in these areas. However, some families find that the development of dementia in one of its members is so traumatising that they need help to address issues that have arisen. Dementia care nurses may work alongside such families by adopting a problem-solving approach (Insert 9:5).

In order to differentiate this approach from methods of assessment that identify people's weaknesses rather than their strengthens, we would highlight that the problem solving approach is concerned

Insert 9:5 A six-point problem-solving strategy for dementia care nursing (adapted from Gamble and Brennan, 2006)

Step 1: What exactly is the problem?
Ask the person with dementia and other family members to say what they think the problem is. Remember that what matters is the family's understanding of the problem rather than yours. Your role is facilitative: to help the family clarify the problem and ensure fair play and equal participation between different family members.

Step 2: List all possible solutions
Ask the family to list different ways in which the problem may be solved. Ask everyone to suggest something. Do not suggest the merits of particular approaches at this stage.

Step 3: Highlight the strengths and advantages
Help the family name the advantages and disadvantages of each suggested solution.

Step 4: Choose the 'best' solution
Encourage the family to discuss and select one particular solution. Help them select a solution that is realistic and achievable.

Step 5: Plan how to carry out the solution
Help the family plan out how they are going to put the suggested solution into action. Help them consider things that may go wrong and anticipate them.

Step 6: Review progress in carrying out homework
Help the family review how 'the solution' was implemented and whether it was successful. Praise effort, rather than achievement. Continue to help the family work on the approach until the situation is fully resolved and well-being promoted.

with the identification of the problem by the family not the nurse and their development of strategies that may resolve the problem.

Sharing the Diagnosis

While it is the role of the medical profession to diagnose dementia, it has been found that a substantial number of GPs do not share the diagnosis with either the person with dementia and/or a family member (Audit Commission, 2000). While there are various reasons why a GP might decide not to share the diagnosis (see Insert 9: 6), Alzheimer Scotland recommends that: 'The benefits of giving the person with dementia the diagnosis, with support and information, mean it is to be recommended in most cases. However, the person with dementia also has a right not to know his or her diagnosis' (www.alzscot.org/pages/policy/righttoknow.htm).

Families do not have a legal right to know the diagnosis and where the person with dementia is not able to give consent, Alzheimer's Scotland (www.alzscot.org/pages/policy/righttoknow.htm) advises that 'it is the responsibility of the doctor to balance the desire or need of the family or carers to know with the rights and best interests of the person with dementia'. They recommend that '[T]o respect the rights of the person with dementia, the diagnosis should normally only be given to the person's family with his or her consent, except in exceptional cases'.

Insert 9:6 To share or not to share the diagnosis of dementia (Alzheimer's Scotland Action on Dementia www.alzscot.org/pages/policy/righttoknow.htm)

The case against giving someone with dementia the diagnosis

- Adverse effect on the person with dementia – possible depression, suicide risk.
- The effect of the illness on the ability to understand, remember take decisions.
- Families' and carers' wish to spare the person with dementia distressing information.
- Medical professionals' uncertainty about the reliability of diagnosis and feelings of helplessness.

The case for giving someone with dementia the diagnosis

- The right to be given medical information in order to maximise autonomy and choice in making informed decisions concerning the future.
- To relieve the anxiety of uncertainty; many people are already aware that something is wrong.
- To avoid paternalistic assumptions, as many people with dementia may cope with the news well.
- Early diagnosis means more people will be able to understand the diagnosis and make choices.
- To avoid a communication barrier between relatives and the person with dementia so that they can be included together in planning for the future.
- Medical professionals' knowledge and feelings are changing due to more precise methods of diagnosis, more information and new and forthcoming treatments.

The *NSF for Older People* (DH, 2001) identifies the importance of the early diagnosis of people with dementia and argues that it enables them to respond effectively to the condition. Manthorpe et al. (2003) found that some nurses already share the diagnosis of dementia with patients while others have the experience and confidence to do so. We would support this finding and suggest that in many clinical settings nurses are often the most appropriate person to disclose the diagnosis to the person with dementia. Nevertheless, we believe that clear guidelines for diagnosis sharing by nurses should be developed and would promote good practice.

Key Principles and Guidelines for Giving the Diagnosis of Dementia

Nurses should discuss the need to disclose the diagnosis with a medical practitioner and other members of the multi-professional team. Disclosing the diagnosis may take a number of meetings. McKillop (2002), who has dementia himself, asserts that 'Being told of the diagnosis at the right time, in the right place, by the right person who has thoughtfully allowed plenty of time for explanations and any questions is essential' (p. 110). Information needs to be given according to the circumstances and receptiveness of the person with dementia and/or carer, with consideration to the background of the person with dementia and their present ability to understand.

Diagnosis-sharing should form part of the information-giving progress that is a key feature of the work undertaken by dementia care nurses. The nurse should choose a suitable place to share the diagnosis that is comfortable and private and has access to support during or after the disclosure from other members of the family where possible. Engagement with the person who has dementia and/or family carer should be underpinned by Rogerian ideas such as those as discussed earlier.

The nurse needs to explore with the person who has dementia how much they know already and how much more they want to know. This is best accomplished by encouraging them to talk about what is happening, employing active listening (and watching) and making inferences about how much they do and do not know and from time to time, checking their understanding. The nurse needs to be careful only to tell the person as much as they want to know and are able to take in. The nurse also needs to find out whether they would like other people to know the diagnosis, for example a particular member of their family or a close friend. If consent has been given that a particular person should know the diagnosis, they then should be told the diagnosis and allowed to attend further meetings, if they and the person with dementia both agree.

The nurse needs to tell the person that they have a type of dementia, say Alzheimer's disease or multi-infarct dementia and briefly explain to them the condition and the implications it will have on their life. Attention should be given to watch the person and observe whether they are displaying any non-verbal signs that they do not want to hear more. The nurse should describe different services that are available in the locality and what they may have to offer. The nurse should display a realistic though positive outlook to the person with dementia that focuses on what they will be able to do, and engenders feelings of hope and promotes a sense of well-being. It may be appropriate for the nurse to discuss issues such as whether they think they should continue driving or whether they require financial and legal help. The nurse should listen and record the views of the person with dementia about the services they would like to have. The nurse should consider, if possible, whether to encourage the person with dementia to identify a formal set of advance directives. The Alzheimer's Society (2001) describes an advance directive as a means whereby a person can give consent on certain treatment or care, refuse certain treatments or nominate someone to do so, on their behalf. An advance directive does not give the person the right to refuse basic care or ask the doctor to do something that is unlawful. The extent of the disclosure should be communicated to other members of the multi-disciplinary team and a written record should be made.

Crisis Work

Nurses should preferably meet people with dementia and their family as soon possible after the onset of the dementia as a means of preventing crisis situations. Sometimes, however, GPs do not refer people with dementia to specialist dementia care services sufficiently early and leads to the eruption of a crisis due to the accumulation of emotional stress in one or more family members.

Insert 9:7 Case example: a crisis waiting to happen

Mr Jackson had dementia and lived in an isolated part of the country in a terraced cottage next to his daughter. He had become increasingly forgetful and confused over the past few years and his daughter looked after him, though it had become increasingly difficult. She often tried to get help for her father from his GP but the GP did not refer Mr Jackson to a psychiatrist. The last straw occurred when a piece of coal shot out from his fireplace and started a small fire in his living room. By chance, his son was working at the local hospital saw the unit for people with dementia, and went in for help. The Sister saw the son and the daughter together, listened to them and helped them work out an action plan. By these means, the daughter and son gained a sense of well-being.

Caplan (1964) identifies three phases of a crisis that may be applied to people giving care to relatives with dementia.

- *Onset*: The immediate increase in tension as the person sees no immediate solution to their problem.
- *Breakdown/recognition*: Tension and anxiety quickly increase and the person's coping strategies become exhausted. At this stage, they may look to others for help and/or stop meeting their responsibilities or cease caring for themselves.
- *Resolution*: Some kind of resolution may occur which may be positive or negative. If the outcome is positive then the person has learnt something worthwhile that may be used in the future and will prevent new ways of coping. Positive outcomes contribute to a person's well-being.

An example of a crisis that arose may be found in the case of Mr Jackson (see Insert 9:7).

Nurses often need to make a quick assessment of clinical situations and this should take place in a calm and thoughtful manner. The formal assessment should preferably occur in the person's home where other family and friends may be present at the time, though the reality is that assessment is usually ongoing. The nurse needs to observe

- *the person experiencing crisis*: whether the person with dementia and/or a family member displays evidence of physical decline such as looking dishevelled, dirty or untidy;

▶ *the person's living environment*: whether there is any evidence of chaotic living;

▶ *evidence of abnormal cognitive or mood state*: whether the person experiencing the crisis is displaying confusion or disorientation or whether they are anxious or depressed;

▶ *physical conditions and disabilities*: whether the person experiencing the crisis has physical conditions and disabilities that may be contributing to the crisis or preventing well-being;

▶ *other people who are present and how they interact with each other*: the nurse needs to look at and listen to the people such as various family members who are in the meeting and see how they are interacting with each other and the person with dementia;

▶ *listening*: the nurse needs to actively listen to the person experiencing crisis. This will not only help the nurse understand the nature of the crisis and enable them to work effectively alongside the person with dementia but will also allow the person in crisis to feel valued and have access to a means of unloading uncomfortable feelings;

▶ *asking questions*: by listening to the person experiencing the crisis, the experienced nurse will be able to find opportunities that will help them express their feelings;

▶ *helping the person identify the difficulty*: by listening and asking questions, the person experiencing the crisis will often come to a better understanding of the essential cause of the crisis;

▶ *developing problem-solving skills*: the nurse can employ a problem-solving approach as described earlier in the chapter. This will not only provide a means of empowerment that will help them resolve the immediate crisis but will also provide an example of how crises may be resolved.

Medication Management

While there is no cure for dementia, various drug treatments have been developed that can slow down the progression of Alzheimer's disease and contribute towards their well-being. These drugs are Aricept, Exelon and Reminyl, which all work in a similar way and are known as acetylcholinesterase inhibitors. There is also a newer drug, Ebixa, which works in a different way to the other three.

Numerous studies have shown that there is depletion in the amount of a chemical called acetylcholine in the synapses in the brains of people with Alzheimer's disease. Acetylcholine is one of the chemicals that nerve cells use to pass messages from one neurone to another.

Aricept, Exelon and Reminyl prevent an enzyme known as acetylcholinesterase from breaking down acetylcholine in the brain. Increased concentrations of acetylcholine lead to increased communication between nerve cells, which may in turn temporarily improve or stabilise the features of Alzheimer's disease.

The action of Ebixa is quite different to, and more complex than, that of Aricept, Exelon and Reminyl. Ebixa blocks the neurotransmitter chemical called glutamate. Glutamate is released in excessive amounts when brain cells are damaged by Alzheimer's disease, which causes the brain cells to be damaged further. Ebixa can protect brain cells by blocking this release of excess glutamate (see Insert 9:8).

What are the Benefits of the Drugs?

It is impossible to predict the potential benefits of using any of these drugs. Some people will improve, some will not, while others will continue to deteriorate. In cases where these drugs prove effective, they appear to slow down the progression of symptoms, including memory loss. They can also improve mood, reduce anxiety and restore confidence.

People who do not show an improvement or slowing down of symptoms in the first few months are unlikely to show any benefit later on. In these cases the drugs will be stopped.

When someone stops taking a drug they are benefiting from, their condition will deteriorate over a period of about four to six weeks until they are no better than someone who has not taken the drug.

Anti-dementia drugs, NICE and Political Action

Discussion of the medication and the effect it has on the experience of the person with dementia should include wider socio-political systems. Many people have difficulty challenging government policy not least, people who have a cognitive impairment and groups are often required to stimulate and challenge government action and policy. At the time of writing (April 2007) a conflict has been raging for the past three years about people's rights to have anti-dementia medication. In March 2005, NICE ruled that drug treatments for dementia should not be prescribed on the NHS

Insert 9.8 Pharmacological Treatments of Alzheimer's disease

Drug	Optimal Client Group	Action	Dose Range	Possible Side Effects
Aricept	Mild to moderate Alzheimer's disease	Acetylcholine-esterase inhibitors	Aricept is taken once a day with or without food. It is available in 5 mg or 10 mg tablets	Nausea and vomiting, diarrhoea, stomach cramps and headaches, dizziness, fatigue, insomnia, loss of appetite.
Exelon	Mild to moderate Alzheimer's disease	Acetylcholine-esterase inhibitors	Exelon is taken twice a day, normally in the morning and evening. People start with 3 mg a day, which will usually increase to a dosage of between 6 mg and 12 mg.	Nausea and vomiting, diarrhoea, stomach cramps and headaches, dizziness, fatigue, insomnia and loss of appetite.
Reminyl	Mild to moderate Alzheimer's disease	Acetylcholine-esterase inhibitors	Reminyl is available as tablets for maintenance treatment (twice-daily 8 mg and 12 mg) and as Reminyl XL once-daily capsules will	Nausea and vomiting, diarrhoea, stomach cramps and headaches, dizziness, fatigue, insomnia and loss of appetite.

| Ebixa | Middle and later stages of Alzheimer's disease | Blocks a messenger chemical, known as a neurotransmitter glutamate. Glutamate is released in excessive amounts when brain cells are damaged by Alzheimer's disease, which causes the brain cells to be damaged further. | continue to be available. Reminyl is available as a 4 mg/ml (twice-daily) oral solution. Ebixa comes in two forms, as 10 mg tablets and as 10 mg oral drops. The tablets can be broken in half into 5 mg doses, and taken with or without food. The recommended starting dose is 5 mg a day, increasing after four weeks to up to 20 mg a day. | Hallucination, confusion, dizziness, headaches and tiredness. Ebixa is not recommended for people with severe kidney problems, but only because there has been no safety test for this group of people yet. Caution is recommended for people with epilepsy and heart problems. |

because of their cost. Following overall condemnation from the public and professions NICE changed its position and allowed limited access to the treatments. However, this meant that still many people with dementia could not have these drugs and in January 2007, the Alzheimer's Society and other organisations lodged a Judicial Review at the High Court. The action taken by these organisations and also thousands of people who have written letters of support, joined marches and publicly supported the position that people with dementia have the right to medication, displays how collective political action is sometimes required to ensure that people with dementia are able to experience optimal recovery. In this way, people with dementia, their families and nurses can use networks to voice what they want at a political level. However, we are aware that political action is also urgently required on a number of other issues of concern to people with dementia such as the quality of care provision in care homes and hospitals and the funding of places in these homes.

Summary

This chapter has examined various activities and interventions that may be used by nurses working with people who have dementia and their families. An initial distinction is made between individual work and family work though it is important to point out that family work should always seek to include the person with dementia. The chapter draws on an activity approach towards older people, that supports the participation of people with dementia in enjoyable and worthwhile activities. The chapter examines various individual and family approaches and interventions that may be used to promote the well-being of people with dementia and their families. These approaches include psychosocial interventions relating to information-giving, crisis intervention and problem solving together with interventions directed towards the management of medication.

References

Allen, K. (2006). Environmental and team approaches to communication in the dementias. In K. Bryan and J. Maxim (eds) *Communication Disability in the Dementias*. London: Whurr, pp. 73–124.

Alzheimer's Society (2001). *Alzheimer's Scotland Action on Dementia*. www.alzscot.org/pages/policy/righttoknow.htm

Audit Commission (2000). *Forget Me Not: Mental Health Services for Older People*. London: Audit Commission.

Baines, S. Saxby, P. and Ehlert, K. (1987). Reality orientation and reminiscence therapy: A controlled cross-over study of elderly confused people. *British Journal of Psychiatry* 151, 22–31.

Ballard, C. G., O'Brien, J., James, I. and Swann, A. (eds) (2001). *Dementia: Management of Behavioural and Psychological Symptoms.* Oxford: Oxford University Press.

Boss, P. (2002). *Family Stress Management* (2nd ed.). London: Sage.

Brooker, D., Snape, M., Johnson, E., Ward, D. and Payne, M. (1997). Single case evaluation of the effects of aromatherapy on disturbed behaviour in senile dementia. *British Journal of Clinical Psychology* 36, 287–296.

Brown, S., Götell, E. and Ekman, S-L. (2001). Singing as a therapeutic intervention in dementia care. *Journal of Dementia Care* July/August, 33–37.

Caplan, G. (1964). *Principles of Preventative Psychiatry.* London: Tavistock.

Clair, A. (2000). The importance of singing with elderly patients. In D. Aldridge *Music Therapy in Dementia Care.* London: Jessica Kingsley Publications, pp. 81–101

Coaten, R. (2001). Exploring reminiscence through dance and movement. *Journal of Dementia Care* 9, 5, 19–22.

Cummings, E. and Henry, W. E. (1961). *Growing old: The process of disengagement.* New York: Basic Books

Davies, S. (2003). Creating community: the basis for caring partnerships in nursing homes. In M. Nolan, U. Lundh, G. Grant and J. Keady (eds) *Partnerships in Family Care: Understanding the Caregiving Career.* Maidenhead: Open University Press, pp. 218–237,

Department of Health (2001). *The NSF for Older People.* London: DH.

Dodds, P. (2007a). Pre-therapy, contact work and dementia care. In P. Sanders (ed) *The Contact Primer.* Ross-on-Wye: PCCS Books, pp. 72–82.

Dodds, P. (2007b). Some considerations on learning and teaching pre-contact reflections In P. Sanders (ed.) *The Contact Primer.* Ross-on-Wye: PCCS Books, pp. 89–101.

Erikson, E. H., Erikson, J. M. and Kivnick, H. Q. (1986). *Vital Involvement in Old Age: The Experience of Old Age in Our Time.* New York: Norton.

Feil, N. (1982). *Validation: The Feil Method.* Cleveland: Feil Productions.

Feil, N. (1993). *The Validation Breakthrough.* Baltimore: Health Professionals Press.

Foth (1999). What is *Art Therapy? Buckeye Art Therapy Association* [brochure] Cleveland OH: Buckeye Art Therapy Association.

Gamble. C. (2006). Building relationships. In C. Gamble and G. Brennan *Working with Serious Mental Illness: A Manual for Clinical Practice.* Edinburgh: Elsevier, pp. 73–83.

Gamble, C. and Brennan, G. (2006). *Working with Serious Mental Illness: A Manual for Clinical Practice*. Edinburgh: Elsevier.

Havighurst, R. J. (1963). Successful Ageing. In R. H. Williams, C. Tibbetts and W. Donahue (eds) *Processes of Aging Volume 1*, New York: Atherton, pp. 299–320.

Holden, W. and Woods, B. (1995). *Positive Approaches to Dementia Care*. Edinburgh: Churchill Livingstone.

Holtkamp, C. C., Kraight, K. van Dongan, M. C., van Rossum, E. and Salentijn, C. (1997). Effects of Snoezelen on the behavior of demented elderly. *Tijdschrift Voor Gerontologie en Geriatrie* 28, 124–128.

Hope, K. (1997). Using multisensory environments with older people with dementia. *Journal of Advanced Nursing* 25, 4, 780–785.

Innes, A. and Hatfield, K. (2001). *Healing Arts Therapies and Person-centred Dementia Care*. London: Jessica Kingsley Publications.

Kahn-Denis, K. B. (2005). Art therapy with geriatric dementia clients. *Art Therapy Journal of American Art Therapy Association* 14, 194–199.

Killick, J. and Allen, K. (2001). *Communication and the Care of People with Dementia*. Buckingham: Open University Press.

Killick, J. and Allen, K. (2005). Good sunset project: quality of life in advanced dementia. *Journal of Dementia Care* 13, 6, pp. 22–23.

Killick, J. and Allen, K. (2006). The getting through initiative: inside the intervention. *Journal of Dementia Care* 14, 2, pp. 27–28.

Kontos, P. C. (2006). Embodied selfhood: the expression of ethnographic of Alzheimer's disease. In A. Leibing and L. Cohen (eds) *Thinking about Dementia: Culture, Loss and the Anthropology of Senility*. New Brunswick: Rutgers University Press, pp. 195–217.

Kitwood, T (1997). *Dementia Reconsidered*. Buckingham: Open University Press.

Kragt, K., Holtkamp, C. C., van Dongan, M. C., van Rossum, E. and Salentijn, C. (1997). The effect of sensory stimulation in the sensory stimulation room on the well-being of demented elderly: A cross-over trial in residents of the R.C. Care Center Bernardus in Amsterdam, *Verpleegkunde* 12, 227–236.

Manthorpe, J., Illiffe, S. and Eden, A. (2003). Early recognition of dementia by nurses. *Journal of Advanced Nursing* 46, 3, 303–310.

McKillop, J. (2002). Did research change anything? In H. Wilkinson (ed.) *The Perspective of People with Dementia*. London: Jessica Kingsley Publications, pp. 109–114.

MacMahon, S. and Kermode, S. (1998). A clinical trial of the effect of aromatherapy on motivational behaviour in dementia care settings using a single subject design. *Australian Journal of Holistic Nursing* 5, 47–49.

Mitchell, S. (1993). Aromatherapy's effectiveness in disorders associated with dementia. *International Journal of Aromatherapy* 5, 20–24.

Nyström, K. and Lauritzen, S. O. (2005). Expressive bodies: demented persons' communication in a dance therapy context. *Health* 9, 3, 297–317.

Osborn, C. (1993). *The Reminiscence Handbook: Ideas for Creative Activities with Older People*. London: Age Exchange.

Pinkney, L. (1997). A comparison of the Snoozlem environment and a music relaxation group on the mood and behaviour of patients with senile dementia. *British Journal of Occupational Therapy* 60, 209–212.

Rogers, C. (1983). *The Freedom to Learn for the 80s*. Columbus OH: Merrill.

Thorgrimsen, L., Spector, A., Wiles, A. and Orrell, M. (2003). Aroma therapy for dementia. In *Cochrane Database of Systematic Reviews* Issue 2, Cochrane review abstract and plan language summary www.Cpcchrane.org.reviews/en/ab/aboo3150.html

Queen-Daugherty, H. (2001). From Heart into Art: person-centred therapy. In Innes, A. and Hatfield, K. (eds) *Healing Arts Therapies and Person-centred Dementia Care*. London: Jessica Kingsley Publications, pp. 19–48.

Victor, C. (2005). *The Social Context of Ageing: A Textbook of Gerontology*. London: Routledge.

Zarit, S. H., Orr, N. and Zarit, J. (1986). *Hidden Victims of Alzheimer's Disease: Families under Stress*. New York: New York University Press.

Chapter 10

Dementia care nursing, emotional labour and clinical supervision

Ingrid Eyers and Trevor Adams

Learning Outcomes

After reading the chapter, you will be able to

- discuss the ideas of emotional labour and body work in relationship to nursing people with dementia;
- evaluate your own emotions experienced when nursing people with dementia;
- develop your own emotional labour tools;
- understand the importance of clinical supervision as a means of preventing emotional labour;
- develop strategies that will help prevent the potential abuse of people with dementia and facilitate person-centred care.

Introduction

Nursing older people with dementia involves a considerable amount of emotional labour (Lee-Treweek, 1996; Eyers, 2000, a, b). This is especially relevant in the provision of care to people with dementia in which it has been identified by Kitwood (1997) that defensive working practices are developed in order to help staff cope with situations that might cause them distress. The importance of emotions in care giving is widely acknowledged (James, 1989, 1992; Smith, 1992; Lee-Treweek, 1996, 1997; Smith and Gray, 2000; Eyers, 2000 a, b, 2007). However, it is an issue that is easily overlooked or taken for granted in the context of nursing people living with dementia. This chapter addresses the issue of emotions experienced by nurses working in dementia care settings and considers the use of emotional labour tools when delivering care, which, in turn, highlights the need for clinical supervision in dementia care nursing.

The tasks involved in meeting the health and social care needs of older people requiring assistance with everyday activities have been classified by Twigg (2000) as 'body work'. This term is used to describe paid work that is related to other people's bodies. Within nursing it is a form of paid work that incorporates not only the physical contact of the nurse with people but also personal and emotional experiences, and the use of 'emotional labour tools' to evoke emotions that will gain the co-operation needed in order to undertake 'body work'. Body work needs to be considered from the perspective of both the care recipient and paid-for carers, such as qualified nurses and health care assistants. Before discussing this issue further, it is important to clarify the concepts of 'body work' and 'emotional labour'.

Body Work

Occupations ranging from health care to the leisure industry are involved in body work and are undertaken by doctors, nurses and personal trainers (Wolkowitz, 2002). The physical tasks in these occupations are related to the human body and often involve direct bodily contact. In nursing, the actual body work undertaken often involves intruding into the very personal and private spheres of older people's lives when they are living with a medical condition that impacts on their everyday life and affects their ability to independently undertake everyday activities that most people take for granted. People who are cognitively impaired are just like anybody else in their need to maintain dignity and privacy and consequently will often reject assistance with very personal tasks. On the other hand, there might be times when their sense of embarrassment is lacking and what is considered by others as inappropriate behaviour occurs. Each of these situations can lead to challenging behaviour that can be emotionally distressing for staff and equally call upon the use of emotional labour tools.

The very personal bodily function of using the toilet to excrete urine and faeces is a situation that often depends on the assistance, guidance or support of a second person. The situation of care staff on such occasions is described by Twigg (2000), who points out that staff providing care to older people in their own home repeatedly identified dealing with 'shit' (*the term used by Twigg in her article*) as difficult, as the smell was hard to bear and had 'an all pervasive, stomach churning quality that lingered about the person' (Twigg, 2000: p. 396). This part of body work may be difficult for nurses but what about its impact upon the dignity and identity of the person with dementia? As this is an area that is not discussed in 'polite society', it has not been easily researched and evaluated from the perspective of the person with dementia. For nurses it is a part of their work, something that is taken for granted and does not merit much discussion. However, such an intrusion into the personal area of bodily functions is an aspect of life that every adult can be expected to empathise with, as it relates to a natural bodily function that we all experience. Whilst coping with incontinence may be unpleasant for nurses, it must surely be perceived as degrading and undignified for the person with dementia.

Much of the body work undertaken in these circumstances is collectively termed as 'basic care' and involves tasks perceived as rudimentary such as washing, dressing and toileting. However, basic care is vital to the well-being of the person with dementia and is an important assessment tool for nurses as it enables them to evaluate both the physical and cognitive well-being of the person for whom they are responsible. This forms an important aspect of short term and long-term care. However, staffing structures are such that vital care is predominantly provided by unqualified nurses and care plans are mainly devised by qualified staff who are often not directly involved in these vital aspects of care.

The division of labour between qualified and unqualified dementia care nurses reproduces the division of labour within nursing that has been identified by Lawler (1991: pp. 30–31) in which nursing is divided into 'basic nursing' and 'technical nursing'. Twigg (2000) describes the hierarchy of care work that is prevalent in body work where unqualified staff undertake the 'dirty work' and the 'clean/technical' tasks are performed by qualified staff. 'Dirty work' is identified as low-status work that is invisible (Lawler, 1991; Lee-Treweek, 1997; Twigg, 2000). Its invisibility is not just because it occurs behind closed doors or screens but because it corresponds to society's perception of traditional female roles in which 'caring is central but poorly valued' (Lawler, 1991: p. 35). Furthermore, women are often perceived to enjoy care work as it is seen to be an extension of their natural role (Lee-Treweek, 1997). This is further emphasised by the invisibility of skills such as informal 'mothering skills' (Ribbens, 1994; Mason, 1996; Williams, 2002), which are taken for granted and brought into formal care giving by a predominantly female workforce. It appears to be assumed that women are naturally equipped to deal with bodily substances encountered in body work and that they are more sympathetic and better able to provide emotional support for others. Body work that is an intrinsic part of care work in dementia care nursing can be seen as physically and emotionally taxing whilst also heavy and dirty. Nursing people with dementia is, at times, concerned with unpleasant body work. As emotional labour and the use of emotional labour tools are employed to undertake body work, this aspect of dementia care nursing is discussed in the next section.

Emotional Labour

Dementia care nursing unavoidably elicits emotions in nurses who are at the same time likely to be implementing emotional labour tools in the provision of care. This exemplifies the dichotomy encountered in emotional labour within health care settings. In the care giving processes of washing and dressing a person, 'emotional labour tools' are used (Eyers, 2006) these can be identified as listening, gentle persuasion, firm direction, discomfort and force (James, 1989: p. 24). In the context of providing care to people with dementia, emotional labour tools are implemented as a means of manipulating an older person into being co-operative so that effective care can be provided within a restricted period of time (Eyers, 2000a, b, 2007). Within formal care giving, time is an important aspect to be addressed. Considering the nature of the emotional labour tools, it becomes clear how their inappropriate use could lead to emotional, physical and verbal abuse.

Hochschild (1983) identifies that in order to survive in a job there is the need to detach oneself mentally from personal feelings that are defined as similar to the sensory experience of hearing or seeing. As exemplified by a participant in a study by Twigg (2000), this also includes smell. To detach oneself from the feeling of revulsion described earlier is something that has to be learned and care assistants are expected to do this through experience at work. Care staff need to learn to detach themselves from emotions such as revulsion or the fear of death, which in health care is not perceived as a good outcome (Lee, 2002).

According to Smith and Gray (2000), student nurses receive guidance and support from mentors and lecturers about how to come to terms with their emotions when they are in direct contact with patients throughout their training. As Hochschild (1983) identifies, care staff need to detach themselves from their own feelings in order to survive in the workplace. However, of all occupations in which emotional labour has been studied, nursing older people with dementia can be seen to be one of the few areas where a long-term interpersonal relationship between the 'service user' and the 'service provider' can arise. Such a long-term relationship can be expected to involve a number of emotions including affection, happiness, frustration, revulsion and sadness. Thus, for new and unqualified nurses in dementia care nursing, an element of fear of not being able to cope with challenging behaviour can also be expected when confronted with situations that are new to them. Here the support and guidance of experienced colleagues is invaluable.

The dichotomy of emotional labour in dementia care nursing can be seen to be related to the fact that whilst nurses are trying to detach themselves from personal emotions, they are also using emotional labour tools. This arises from the requirement to meet the care needs of the people nurses are employed to care for within a tight time schedule (James, 1989; Lee-Treweek, 1997; Eyers, 2000 a, b, 2007; James, 1989).

Emotional labour can be seen as demanding skilled work, as it is about 'action and reaction, doing and being' (James, 1992: p. 500). James defines it as 'the labour involved in dealing with other people's feelings, a core component of which is the regulation of emotions' (James, 1989: p. 15). In dementia care nursing, emotional labour tools are implemented as a means of manipulating an older person into being co-operative in order to undertake body work in the shortest possible time (Eyers, 2000a, 2006). As described earlier the 'emotional tools' used in care comprise listening, gentle persuasion, firm direction, discomfort and force (James, 1989: p. 24), and represent a further development of Hochschild's (1983) seminal work on emotional labour.

Emotional labour is perceived by Hochschild (1983) to be better understood and used by women. She asserts that:

> In general, lower-class and working-class people tend to work more with things, and middle-class and upper-class people tend to work more with people. More working women than men deal with people as a job. Thus there are both gender patterns and class patterns to the civic and

commercial use of human feelings. That is the social point. (Hochschild, 1983: p. 21)

The established low status of body work indicates how health care services such as nursing use gender differences to their advantage but do not acknowledge the commercial value of such a gender difference. Women who are able to facilitate and order emotions are of interest to nursing services, as such attributes keep customers happy and women's emotional labour skills have become a saleable low-priced commodity within the public sphere (Lee-Treweek, 1996). The importance of this gender difference established by Hochschild (1983) is further researched within the health-care sector by Smith (1992), Smith and Gray (2000), James (1989, 1992) and Lee Treweek (1996).

The work of Smith (Smith 1992; Smith and Gray 2000) focuses predominantly on emotional labour and student nurse training and highlights the importance of acknowledging the role of emotions within hospital work. James (1989, 1992) based her study on hospice care and identified the use of emotional labour tools that are developed throughout a person's life and through their experience of care work. This study has been expanded by Lee-Treweek (1996) who undertook an ethnographic study of staff in residential care homes in which she observed how order was created through kindness, nurturance and knowledge (Lee-Treweek, 1996: p. 120). The relationship between older people and care staff is seen as reciprocal, intimate and mimicking family bonds (Lee-Treweek, 1996; Caris-Verhallen, 1999). Smith and Gray (2000) also report how student nurses referred to family relationships when relating their feelings about their experiences nursing hospital patients. This indicates how emotional labour skills developed within the personal family could be transferred to the work-place 'family'. However, this skill transferral calls for supervision and guidance when new staff are learning to cope with situations they have never previously encountered. Staff learn from one another and are not always fully aware of the appropriate use of emotional labour tools. Indeed they are unlikely to realise that they are using emotional labour tools, unless this has been brought to their attention and discussed.

The outcome of emotional labour depends on how skilfully the paid-for carers deal with encountered situations (James, 1992). The constraints experienced by paid-for carers are compared to those of a factory worker, as in each case it is about process and order.

Health care assistants are seen to produce a clean, orderly, quiet care recipient without too much thought or personal input. Knowing the older person equates to knowing one's materials in the manufacturing process, and health care assistants consider their 'product knowledge' to be superior to that of the qualified nurse working alongside them. Care work has been described as an ongoing production process rather than as a set of person-centred acts (Lee-Treweek, 1997). Despite the rhetoric of person-centred care, the reality of care work is determined by the contact time potentially available between care giver and care recipient (Eyers, 2007). Owing to the conflict between 'process time' (the actual time need to complete a task thoroughly) and 'clock time' (the actual time available) body work is undertaken using emotional labour tools in order to shorten the process time and to be seen to be competent to work within the available clock time (Eyers, 2007). For example, a health care assistant may have six people to wake up, wash and dress within two hours. That means on average there are 20 minutes available per person. However, it might take longer than that to wash and dress someone who has been doubly incontinent and is presenting challenging behaviour. The 'clock time' in this instance would be 20 minutes but the 'process time' could well be 30 minutes. The additional 10 minutes are taken away from the next person who is hopefully compliant, and with the use of product knowledge and appropriate use of emotional labour tools to positively encourage co-operation, work can be completed in the remaining time. Unqualified nurses are constantly working within such time constraints, and such a conflict can be seen to jeopardise the implementation of person-centred care. Feelings of guilt and inadequacy are potentially added to the emotions experienced by dementia care nurses initially wanting to provide the best possible care.

Care Giving

A range of emotions experienced by care staff, including nurses, has been considered in the context of care giving. At times, challenging behaviour can be displayed unexpectedly by older people with dementia and this can evoke elements of fear and possible physical pain. In these situations, knowledge and understanding of the cause of such behaviour will ease the strength of those emotions. This forms part of the set of formally acquired coping strategies. Emotional labour can be seen as demanding skilled work, as it is about 'action and reaction, doing and being' (James, 1992, p. 500).

Without adequate training to cope with challenging behaviour, dementia care nurses will develop their own coping mechanisms that may not always be suitable for either the nurse or the client.

As Hochschild (1983) and Kitwood (1997) have identified, nurses tend to detach themselves from their own feelings in order to survive in the workplace. As Kitwood and Bredin (1992) note: "Professionals and informal carers are vulnerable people too, bearing their own anxiety and dread concerning frailty, dependence, madness, ageing, dying and death. A supposed objectivity in a context that is, in fact, interpersonal is one way of maintaining psychological defences, and so making involvement with conditions such as dementia bearable." (p. 270)

The emotional attachments that can be established in dementia care need to be acknowledged and respected. How paid-for carers deal with emotional labour, interact and maintain optimal engagement with older people they care for is likely to be determined by their understanding of the complex needs of people living with a long-term condition such as dementia.

Clinical Supervision

Nursing people with dementia and their families is physically and emotionally demanding and calls for the skilled use of emotional labour tools. Working alongside older people with dementia will frequently result in nurses using emotionally protective practices that distance themselves from the person with dementia and will lead to impaired therapeutic engagement. As a means of reducing these practices and also increasing therapeutic engagement between nurses and people with dementia, we would recommend that clinical supervision should be an essential feature of dementia care nursing and employing authorities should offer regular and paid clinical supervision to all dementia care nurses.

Clinical supervision has been defined within the context of nursing as 'a formal process of professional support and learning which enables individual practitioners to develop knowledge and competence, assume responsibility for their own practice and enhance consumer protection and safety of care in complex situations' (DH, 1993). Clinical supervision initially developed outside nursing, within psychotherapy. While Emmerton (1999) argues that supervision formed part of the legacy gained from Florence Nightingale, clinical supervision was first discussed in relationship to nursing in the USA in the 1950s. Interest in clinical supervision as a component of nursing did not develop in the United Kingdom until the late 1980s and early 1990s, mainly through the work of Butterworth and Faugier (1994) who see it as an exchange between practising professionals that enables the development of professional skills. The 1994 governmental review on Mental Health Nursing entitled *Working in Partnership* (DH, 1994) affirmed clinical supervision as an essential feature of mental health nursing. The position of clinical supervision in mental health nursing was reiterated in *From Values to Action* (DH, 2006: p. 39), which suggested that one means of attaining its Recommendation 16 that 'All MHN (mental health nurses) will continue to develop skills and knowledge throughout their career' is for all mental health nurses 'to engage in regular clinical supervision from suitably trained supervisors and this process to be audited'. Within this context it is also important to consider the needs of health care assistants who experience very little training to help them understand the challenging behaviour they may encounter when aiming to provide vital care to the best of their ability.

There have been only a few studies on the effectiveness of clinical supervision in dementia care nursing. However, the few studies that have been undertaken suggest that it would facilitate good practice. In one study, Graham (1999) interviewed six community mental health nurses receiving regular clinical supervision and working with people who have dementia and their family members. He gave encouraging indications that the clinical supervision these nurses received enhanced their provision of dementia care. More specifically he found indications that clinical supervision encouraged the nurses to implement person-centred care and promoted good relationships between the nurses and people with dementia and their family members. He found that the clinical supervision increased the interpersonal ability and emotional competence of the nurses and encouraged them to develop helpful insights into the relationship between the person with dementia, their family and the rest of society, and helped the nurses experience lower levels of stress, thus indicating that dealing with personal emotions also contributes to the honing of an individual set of emotional labour tools.

A number of studies undertaken at the University of Lund, Sweden, examine the use of clinical supervision within dementia care nursing. Berg (2000) used data gained from interviews taken on a quasi-experimental study of nurses that had individual and group supervision while working with people who have dementia; the study found that the nurses searched for meaning in their work and that clinical supervision lowered the nurses' experience of burnout and enhanced their creativity.

Various approaches towards clinical supervision have been advocated and can be used with nurses working alongside people with dementia and their families. The approach taken in this book follows that of Brennan and Gamble (2006) who argue that the relationship between the supervisor and supervisee is like that between the client and the practitioner and draws upon Pepleu's model of interpersonal relationships. In addition, Brennan and Gamble (2006) employ a model of reflection developed by Boud et al. (1985) which is used to understand the ways in which different experiences encountered by the supervisee may be turned into learning (see Insert 10.1).

Insert 10:1 Reflection: turning experience into learning (taken from Boud et al. 1985 and Brennan and Gamble, 2006)

Experience
- Behaviour
- Ideas
- Feelings

The reflective process
- Returning to experience
- Utilising positive feelings/attitudes
- Removing negative feelings by processing
- Re-evaluating experience

Outcomes/action
- New perspectives
- New knowledge
- Change in behaviour
- Readiness to put knowledge into practice

Orientation: During this period the nurse and the supervisor meet each other and decide whether they will be able to work together within the context of clinical supervision. It is important that each party has a shared understanding of the nature of clinical supervision and an agreement has been made about what will happen in future sessions.

Identification: The nurse decides what they would like help with and how that help should be given. This is negotiated and agreed with the supervisor. (See Insert 10:2).

Insert 10:2 Orientation and identification within
clinical supervision in dementia care nursing
(adapted from Brennan and Gamble, 2006)

Introduce the models of supervision
Why are you both here?
What do you want to get out of supervision?

Explore dementia care nurse's previous experience of clinical supervision
Did the nurse have any?
Did the nurse have useful supervision from which you can both learn?
Did the nurse have supervision that they found of little use or harmful and from which
you can both learn?

Clarify purpose and expectation
What can supervisor offer?
What does the nurse need to address?

Direct supervisee in goal setting
What, if any, are the clinical needs of the dementia care nurse?

Deal with administration
Who will organise the venue, frequency, note-keeping of meetings?

Exploitation

The nurse and the supervisor then embark on the clinical supervision. The meetings are based on the idea of a collaborative partnership. They are time limited and a time should be agreed when the clinical supervision sessions will be evaluated and whether agreements have been kept. The proceedings of the meeting should be written down and should include a summary of the supervisor's objectives, administrative responsibilities of each party, what happened in the meeting and date for next meeting. The notes should be jointly written and jointly signed.

The purpose of each clinical supervision meeting is to help the dementia care nurse to implement nursing care. During the meeting the supervisor will ask the nurse how they are implementing care to particular people with dementia and their family members or talk about the care they provide to people with dementia and their families as a whole. Using the model of reflection developed by Boud et al. (1985) the supervisee will ask the nurse to talk about behaviour, ideas and feelings they have encountered within specific dementia care settings as a means of helping them discuss, reflect and learn from the situation. The supervisor will help the nurse focus on positive emotions and attitudes they have experienced in the situation and help remove negative emotions in order to re-evaluate the nurse's experience.

Resolution

At the end of the supervision meeting, both the nurse and the supervisor have the opportunity to evaluate what has happened in the meeting, say goodbye and move on in a healthy way. Both parties should be aware of the initial aims and objectives of the supervision and evaluate whether or not they have been accomplished. The supervisor should reaffirm their continued commitment to the supervision process.

Jasper (2006) argues that 'clinical supervision' is a misunderstood term and that the term and its underlying concepts have been manipulated. This manipulation is seen by Jasper (2006) to have led to misunderstandings which may lead to a contravention of the rights of staff. Consequently, the suggestion is that while clinical supervision should be offered to all dementia care nurses it should only be given following a full explanation to the nurse and the nurse's consent. Moreover, should at any time the nurse want to leave clinical supervision they should be allowed to do so. Managerial power should not enforce clinical supervision but rather encourage its beneficial effect on nursing practice and the emotional well-being of the nurse.

An additional complication which leads to further misunderstanding is that 'clinical supervision' has been used to describe many different types of managerial and educational meetings with nurses. As a means of differentiating 'clinical supervision' from various other clinical support meetings that take place between supervisors and managers and different types of nurses, Brennan and Gamble (2006) argue that the distinctive feature of clinical supervision is the lack of control managers have, or should have, over the meeting. Whereas some professions, such as midwifery, think that clinical supervision should comprise professional monitoring, it could be argued that this limits the effectiveness of the supervision and impedes the free exploration and expression of ideas in the meeting. Insert 10.3 outlines the type and nature of different forms of clinical support that are described by Brennan and

Insert 10:3 Five types of educational and clinical support structures (adapted from Brennan and Gamble, 2006)

	Who sets the agenda	Level of confidentiality	Record keeping	Information giving and advice	Challenging the supervisee	Level of support	Level of catalytic help
Clinical supervision	Supervisee	Total, except in the case of legal requirements	Supervision agreement or contract. Contract agreed by the supervisee. Record of attendance and content	Given to supplement supervisees' own expertise to enable them to see own options and make own decisions	Based on evidence given during the supervision session	Supervisee encouraged to recognise and use own expertise. No practical help given outside session	Establishing reflection on issues affecting practice. Planning, decision-making and reviewing
Management supervision	Line manager or delegated other	Not confidential	May be recorded by manager in personal life	Given to direct supervisee towards set objectives or training needs	Based on evidence gained/observed in work situation	Practical help may be given outside session	Manager elicits information on work done and standards achieved
Personal developments review	Organisational policy or document	Not confidential	Copy of PDR. Portions may be sent to other	Given to direct worker towards PDR objectives	Based on evidence gained/observed in work situation	Practical help may be given outside session	Overall performance review and

						objective setting
Disciplinary interview	Investigating manager	Not confidential	organisational departments e.g., to access training Recorded by manager in personal file	Given to instruct and inform worker of the process and possible outcomes	Based on evidence gained/observed in work situation	Practical help may be given outside session or this may be delegated to an independent adviser	Manager elicits information on the issues under discussion and goals
Educational mentoring	The mentor in consultation with the student nurse	Not confidential	Recorded in mentor's and students' notes.	The mentor asks questions that allow the nurses to reflect on their knowledge and feelings about specific situations	Based on evidence gained/observed in work situation and the application of more generalisable theory	Advice may be given within and outside the session including references to peer reviewed papers, text books and course work	Teacher elicits information on the issues under discussion and goals

Gamble (2006). In addition, the table adds mentoring as a form of educational supervision.

While it is important to differentiate clinical supervision from other supportive activities, various forms of educational and clinical support structures may also be seen to address people's experience of emotional labour within dementia care nursing.

Summary

This chapter acknowledges an invisible, intangible yet very important part of nursing which is often overlooked or taken for granted. Coping with the dichotomy of personal emotions ranging from fun to fear whilst constantly using emotional labour tools to provide care within a restrictive time frame underpins the importance of clinical support so that vulnerable older people are able to experience person-centred care. Nursing people with dementia incorporates undertaking vital everyday body work that enhances the quality of life experienced by someone with dementia or participating in activities that can be fun or challenging. In addition, the chapter has described the use of clinical supervision as a means of reducing nurse's experience of emotional labour and promoting their well-being. Understanding and valuing this aspect of nursing not only enhances the well-being of the nurse but also the person with dementia themselves and their families.

References

Berg, A. (2000). Psychiatric nurses' view of nursing care, clinical supervision and individualised care. Interventions on a dementia and on a general psychiatric ward. http://lu-research.lub.lu.se/php/gateway.php?who=lr&method=getfile&file=archive/00009355/

Boud, D. Keogh, R. and Walker, D. (eds) (1985). *Reflection: Turning Learning into Experience*. London: Kogan Page.

Butterworth, T. and Faugier, J. (1994). *Clinical Supervision and Mentorship in Nursing*. London: Chapman Hall.

Caris-Verhallen, W., Kerkstra, A. and Bensing, J. (1999). 'Non-verbal behaviour in nurse-elderly patient communication'. *Journal of Advanced Nursing* 29(4), 808–818.

Department of Health (1993). *Vision for the Future: The Nursing, Midwifery and Health Visiting Contribution to Health and Social Care*. London: HMSO.

Department of Health (2006). *From Values of Action*. London: DH.

Department of Health (1994). *Working in Partnership: A Collaborative Approach to Care*. Report of the Mental Review Team. London: HMSO.

Emmerton, A. Florence Nightingale Memorial Service, Westminster Abbey. London.

Eyers, I. (2000a). Care assistants overlooked? A cross-national study of care home staff in England and Germany. *Quality in Ageing – Policy, Practice and Research* 1(1), 15–26.

Eyers, I. (2000b). Education and Training. Do they really, really want it? A comparative study of care home staff in England and Germany. *Education and Ageing* 15(2), 159–175.

Eyers, I. (2006). Extracting the Essence of Formal Caregiving: A Comparative Study of Formal Care Givers in English and German Care Homes. In Paoletti (ed.) *Family Caregiving to Older Disabled People: Relational and Institutional Issues.* New York, USA: Novascience, pp. 273–294.

Gamble, C. and Brernnan, G. (2006). Working with serious mental illness: a manual for clinical practice (2nd Edition) Edinburgh: Elsevier.

Graham, I. (1999). Reflective narrative and dementia care. *Journal of Clinical Nursing* 8, 6, pp. 675–683(9).

Hochschild, A. R. (1983). *The Managed Heart: Commercialization of Human Feeling.* Berkeley: University of California Press.

James, N. (1989). Emotional labour: skill and work in the social regulation of feelings. *Sociological Review* 37(1), 15–42.

James, N. (1992). Care = organisation + physical labour + emotional labour. *Sociology of Health and Illness* 14(4), 488–509.

Jasper, M. (2006). *Beginning Reflective Practice.* Cheltenham: Nelson Thornes.

Kitwood, T. (1997). *Dementia Reconsidered: The Person Comes First.* Buckingham: Open University Press.

Kitwood, T. and Bredin (1992). Towards a theory of dementia care: personhood and well-being. *Ageing and Society* 12, pp. 268–287.

Lawler, J. (1991). *Behind the Screens. Nursing, Somology, and the Problems of the Body* Edinburgh: Churchill, Livingstone.

Lee, G. (2002). Emotional labour and cancer work: some reflections after a conference. *Soundings* 20, 144–149.

Lee-Treweek, G. (1996). Emotion work, order and emotional power in care assistant work. In V. James and J. Gabe (eds) *Health and the Sociology of Emotions.* Oxford: Blackwell Publishers, pp. 115–132.

Lee-Treweek, G. (1997). Women resistance and care; an ethnographic study of nursing auxiliary work. *Work, Employment and Society* 11(1), 47–63.

Mason, J. (1996). Gender, care and sensibility in family and kin relationships. In J. Holland and L. Adkins (eds) *Sex, Sensibility and the Gendered Body.* Basingstoke: MacMillan, pp. 15–36.

Ribbens, J. (1994). *Mothers and their Children*. London: Sage.

Smith, P. (1992). *The Emotional Labour of Nursing*. Basingstoke: Macmillan.

Smith, P. and Gray, B. (2000). *The Emotional Labour of Nursing: How Student and Qualified Nurses Learn to Care: A Report on Nurse Education, Nursing Practice and Emotional Labour in the Contemporary NHS*. London: South Bank University, Faculty of Health.

Twigg, J. (2000). Carework as a form of bodywork. *Ageing and Society* 20(4), 389–411.

Williams, C. (2002). *Mothers, Young People and Chronic Illness*. Aldershot: Ashgate

Wolkowitz, C. (2002). The social relations of body work. *Work, Employment and Society* 16(3), 497–510.

Chapter 11

Clinical settings, competencies and skills in dementia care nursing

Trevor Adams

Learning Outcomes

After reading the chapter, you will be able to

▶ describe different settings in which dementia care nursing takes place;
▶ describe various capabilities that nurses require to work with people who have dementia and their families;
▶ discuss the relationship between competencies, capabilities, theory and practice;
▶ outline a range of competences and capabilities that nurses require to work with people who have dementia, their families and members of multi-professional and multi-agency teams.

Introduction

This chapter examines the work undertaken by nurses as they promote the well-being of people with dementia and their families. Initially the chapter looks at different settings in which dementia care nursing takes place such as acute, mental health and community settings, including private nursing homes. The chapter continues by looking at the competencies and capabilities that nurses should possess as they work alongside people with dementia and their families. The chapter does this by adapting *The Ten Essential Shared Capabilities for Mental Health Practice* (NIMHE, 2004 and *Best Practice Competencies and Capabilities for Pre-registration Mental Health Nurses in England* (DH, 2006) to dementia care nursing.

Dementia Care Settings

Nurses work alongside people with dementia in different care settings. *From Values to Action* (DH, 2006) says that mental health nurses are best employed working with complex cases and understands complex cases as in working with people in the latter stages of dementia (p. 24). We would suggest that this understanding of 'complexity' is far too narrow and that its use in relationship to dementia care nursing is misleading. We believe that complexity does not merely occur in the latter stages of dementia but is a continuous feature throughout people's experience of dementia. All aspects of a person's dementia, whether it is in its early or latter stages may give rise to complex and difficult situations that require skilled nursing care. We would argue that dementia care nurses have a legitimate and important role throughout the whole course of a person's dementia and that complexity is not merely confined to its latter stages.

Early Intervention

Recent Government policy highlights the need for the early recognition and intervention with people who have dementia. This policy has arisen against a background of medical developments in diagnosis and pharmacology that has led to the reduction of symptoms in Alzheimer's disease (DH, 2005; NAO, 2007). Dementia care nurses have an important role in the early stages of dementia and we would support *Rights, Relationships and Recovery* (Scottish Executive, 2006), which argues that '[M]ental health nurses also provide education and counselling support to families and carers, particularly in the early stages of dementia' (p. 31). We would see this work as promoting the well-being of people with dementia and their families. While this work differs from family to family, it often includes crisis intervention, diagnosis-sharing, information-giving, emotional support and networking.

One type of service that offers early contact with the person who has dementia and their family are services concerned with outreach or assertive management (Cantley and Caswell, 2007). Many people with dementia and their families do not know where to find help and have considerable difficulty looking for appropriate professional support. Sometimes this may be due to services not making themselves known or sometimes it may be due to General Practitioners delaying referral to specialist mental health services for older people in the misbelief that nothing can be done. *From Values to Action* (DH, 2006) supports the need for equal and accessible services for older people with mental health conditions, and to address this issue we would suggest that, where possible, dementia care nurses should adopt 'case finding' approaches to gain new referrals that are unknown to specialist dementia care services.

Another type of service that has developed for people in the early stages of dementia are memory clinics (Lindesay et al., 2002). Their work usually includes offering people a diagnosis of dementia following a range of physical and psychological tests; the prescription and administration of medication that will slow cognitive impairment; pre- and post-diagnostic counselling about the implications of having dementia; and referral to other agencies that may be helpful and supportive. Various types of memory clinic exist; though most are usually based in a hospital setting, the service based at Wythenshawe Hospital, Greater Manchester, is located in the community (Page, 2003).

A further service, that may also provide help and support to people in the early stages of dementia and their families are Alzheimer's Cafés. These services offer a café location in which people with dementia and their close family members can meet other people with dementia and their family carers and find out how it feels to have or care for somebody with dementia (Capus, 2005). Alzheimer's Cafés correspond well with the whole systems approach developed in this book as they allow people with dementia and their relatives to make helpful links with different dementia-orientated agencies in the community. We would see nurses having an important role in the development and maintenance of Alzheimer's Cafés and this includes listening to people's stories; sharing their own story of their own relatives with dementia; promoting learning about dementia; and making cups of tea and cleaning up – why should all the dirty work be done by the volunteers!

Acute General Care

Everybody's Business (DH, 2005) affirms that '[o]lder people with mental health problems in the general hospital have the same right to appropriate care as people outside hospital' (p. 41). The needs of people with dementia in general hospitals often go unrecognised and there is a need for acute services to be 'dementia-friendly'

(Silverstein and Maslow, 2006). Borbasi et al. (2006) in a study on nursing people with dementia in acute general settings found that first, environmental factors often place constraints on ensuring good practice with people who have dementia on acute general wards and are often associated with ensuring their safety on ward areas. Second, some staff may not be sympathetic to nursing people with dementia such as nurses on surgical wards and also younger staff. Third, lack of time and equipment is frequently a constraint and often clinical areas are not dementia-friendly. As *Everybody's Business* (DH, 2005) notes 'the longer the older person stays in an acute bed, the more disorientated they may become, the more independent living skills are lost, and attempts at rehabilitation are lost'. (p. 41)

Securing equal access to mental health services for older people in general hospital settings is a considerable problem (Royal College of Psychiatrists, 2005) and various ways of addressing this issue are suggested in *Everybody's Business* (DH, 2005). (see Insert 11: 1)

A recent study by Nolan (2006) supports the development of person-centred and relationship-centred approaches with people

---

Insert 11:1 Ways of promoting equal access to specialist dementia services to people in acute general care settings (taken from *Everybody's Business* (DH, 2005)

- Mental health teams should work proactively and collaboratively with general hospital teams and raise awareness of the importance of mental health to integrate care within a general hospital setting,
- There should be an improvement in the knowledge, skills and attitudes of all professionals through training programmes and promotion of routine assessment during the admission of all older people at admission,
- Protocols for the management of uncomplicated mental health problems with guidance should improve the general appropriateness of referrals. Protocols should help support and supervise general care teams deal with common mental health conditions,
- Mental health teams should be quick to respond to requests for assessment or advice from general hospital teams on older people with dementia who present themselves in Accident and Emergency Departments, including cases where there is co-morbidity,
- Good discharge planning should exist for older people with dementia
  - through discharge co-ordination teams;
  - regular interface and discussion between senior clinicians on mental health teams and teams within general hospitals.

who have dementia in acute settings. She argues that nurses consider the lives of people with dementia as being meaningful and that lucidity and communication are possible through participatory caring. She highlights the importance of respecting personhood in dementia care and that relationships are the medium through which care is demonstrated and experienced. Similarly, Norman (2006) found that meaningful care for the older person with dementia in the acute settings requires a respectful connection with the patient as a person, through the development of a bond. The meaning of the caring experience was found to relate to the personhood of both the nurse and the patient, experienced within the context of relationship. To make this connection it was necessary to work with relatives and carers who know the patient best.

Middle Stages of Dementia

People in the 'middle' stages of dementia may receive support from a number of agencies, such as families, friends, health services, social services, voluntary agencies and private agencies. Its primary aim is to maintain people with dementia in their own home for as long as possible. Following the provision of services in the early stages of dementia, other services will be required to support the person with dementia and reduce the stress their relatives may be experiencing. These services may include day hospital care for people with dementia; respite care providing residential support for people with dementia for a limited time; relative support groups that offer information and emotional support for relatives of people with dementia. Throughout this period, the attention of the nurse should be on promoting the physical, psychological and social well-being of the person with dementia and their family.

CMHNs often have an important role to play at this stage of the development of dementia, and may undertake a range of approaches such as information-giving, supportive counselling and emotional support, networking and monitoring (Adams, 1996). *Rights, Relationships and Recovery* (Scottish Executive, 2006) outlines a role for mental health nurses that is applicable to nurses working with people who have dementia who have not got a specialist knowledge of mental health care.

Much of the care offered to people with dementia in care home settings is provided by care staff or general nurses. There are opportunities to continue to support and enhance this important area of care through enabling staff in this sector to access mental health nurses' knowledge, skills and experience for clinical advice, education and support.

The CMHN offers a link between the person with dementia, their informal carer(s) and other agencies and services in the community, including the hospital. The CMHN often plays a useful role in the co-ordinating and juggling of scarce services.

Latter Stages of Dementia

As the dementia progresses, the person with dementia will become increasingly physically dependent and an important part of the work of nurses will be to promote not only their emotional well-being but also their physical well-being. The importance of palliative care to people with dementia and its implications has been recently elaborated in the document *Exploring Palliative Care for People with Dementia* (NCPC/Alzheimer's Society, 2006). Albinsson and Strang (2003) identify differences between staff working with people in the latter stages of dementia and staff in palliative care, particularly relating to provision of support at and following the time of death. They found that nurses working with people in the latter stages of dementia tend to be less focused on the client and more focused on the family. Addington-Hall (2000) argues that this gives rise to barriers relating to integrating people with dementia within a hospice environment. However, collaboration has now been proposed between mental health and palliative care services (de Vries, 2003), and it has been shown that multidisciplinary work between palliative care teams and mental health teams for older people teams can have a positive impact on the end-of-life care for people with dementia (Lloyd-Williams and Payne, 2002). Abbey (2003) sets palliative nursing care of people with dementia within a framework that acknowledges the person with dementia and their close family members and asserts the need for shared decision-making on issues such as nutrition, pain relief and different areas of daily living (Henderson, 2007).

Nursing Capabilities and Competencies

We have already noted that nursing people with dementia and their families is a practical activity that it is concerned with what nurses do and say. Recently, agencies such as the Department of Health (2006) have used ideas such as 'capability' and 'competency' to clarify what nurses do. 'Competence' according to Fraser and Greenwood (2001) is what 'individuals know or are able to do in terms of knowledge, skills and attitudes', and different competencies have been identified that are considered should be possessed by all practising dementia care nursing (Mace, 2005). The idea of 'competency' is helpful, though it fails to link competencies with theoretical frameworks that underpin practice. We would argue that the idea of competency is meaningless without it being connected to a specific body of ideas, and that the different competencies that are used depends on the theory that underpins it – the competencies for nurses using a behavioural approach are different from nurses using a psychodynamic approach. Butterworth (1986) argues that in the absence of a theoretical basis to their practice mental health nurses will find themselves under the control of the dominant ideology within health care teams. This is usually the medical model, though it may also be an exclusively psychological model. We would, therefore, suggest that those nurses whose practice is defined by competencies alone will have few ideas to guide, direct and define their practice and will find themselves losing their professional autonomy and increasingly will come under the control of other professions within the multi-professional mental health team.

A more satisfactory idea is 'capability' which is the 'extent to which an individual can apply, adapt and synthesise new knowledge from experience and so continue to improve their performance' (Fraser and Greenwood, 2001). This is a more dynamic and reflexive understanding of nursing practice that while still understands nursing as a practical activity, sees knowledge as arising out of clinical settings.

The Department of Health (2001) has developed ten essential shared capabilities they believe should be possessed by all mental health practitioners. Their purpose is to establish the minimum requirements or capabilities mental health care staff should possess on completion of training. While these capabilities do not specifically relate to either nursing or work with people who have dementia, they do provide a helpful means of identifying important skills that are required by nurses working with people who have dementia and providing a much needed link between mental health nursing for older people and mental health nursing for people of working age.

Ten Essential Capabilities and their Application to Dementia Care Nursing

Working in Partnership: Developing and maintaining constructive working relationships with service users, carers, families, colleagues, lay people and wider community networks; and working positively without tensions created by conflicts of interest or aspiration that may arise between the partners in care.

Nurses working with people who have dementia need to develop good relationships and work alongside everyone involved in the care and support of the person with dementia. To facilitate best practice, nurses need to develop good listening skills and be attuned not just to the voice of the more fluent and able but also to those who have speech impairment as a result of having dementia. Nurses need to hear their story about what has happened and their opinions about what they want. They also need clear and easily understood information and may need help to make decisions.

Respecting Diversity: Working in partnership with service users, carers, families and colleagues to provide care and interventions that not only make a positive difference but also do so in ways that respect and value diversity including age, race, culture, disability, gender, spirituality and sexuality.

Nurses working with people who have dementia need to be sensitive to people with dementia and their families from different cultural backgrounds. Nurses should possess a degree of cultural competence in relation to people with dementia from different cultures (McKenzie et al., 2007). Services should be culture-friendly and should not be off-putting to local community groups that do not share the dominant cultural values and practices. In addition, nurses should recognise the differences between families with respect to age, race and sexuality and nurses working alongside people with dementia should respect these differences.

Practising Ethically: Recognising the rights and aspirations of service users and their families, acknowledging power differentials and minimising them whenever possible; and providing treatment and care that is accountable to service users and family members within the boundaries prescribed by professional, legal and local codes of ethical practice.

Nurses working with people who have dementia should respect the rights and wishes of all those providing dementia care, including people with dementia who may well have an impaired ability to make choices and put their views forward. Differences in power between people with dementia and other members of their family should be fully recognised and minimised by nurses. Nurses working alongside people with dementia are accountable to all users, that is, people with dementia and family members and should fit within legal frameworks, the *'Nurses and Midwifery Code of Practice'* (NMC, 2004) together with relevant codes of ethical practice. While family carers do themselves use services, it is not helpful to identify them as users, as this takes away the right of the person with dementia to be regarded as users.

Challenging Inequality: Addressing the causes and consequences of stigma, discrimination, social inequality and exclusion of service users, carers and mental health services; and creating, developing or maintaining valued social roles for people in the communities they come from.

Nurses working with people who have dementia should address the causes and consequences of stigma, discrimination, social inequality and exclusion with regard to people who have dementia, their family members and dementia care services. These factors constitute 'excess disability' and are due to barriers society places against people with dementia which they find difficult to overcome. Nurses should adopt an advocacy approach to help people with dementia overcome interpersonal and social barriers that disempowers and sets limits on access to services.

Promoting Well-being: Working in partnership to provide care and treatment that enables service users and carers to tackle mental health problems with hope and optimism and to work towards a valued lifestyle within and beyond the limits of any mental health problem.

Nurses working with people who have dementia should help promote the 'well-being' of people with dementia and their families. We would argue that nurses should draw on ways of communication that enable people with dementia to make their views known and allow them to enter into decision-making processes. We would also support nurses making arrangements for people with dementia to take part in purposeful activities that allow them to creatively express themselves and affirm their personhood within social groups of which they are a part.

Identifying People's Needs and Strengths: Working in partnership to gather information to agree health and social care needs in the context of the preferred lifestyle and aspirations of service users, their families, carers and friends.

Nurses working with people who have dementia should assess different bodily and social systems – biological, family, social and socio-political – that interact with each other. Within this systemic framework, the respective strengths of the person with dementia and also different members of their family and friends should be highlighted. These strengths should be linked to local strengths within service provision and incorporated within a nursing care plan.

Providing Service User-Centred Care: *Negotiating achievable and meaningful goals; primarily from the perspective of service users and their families. Influencing and seeking the means to achieve these goals and clarifying the responsibilities of the people who will provide any help that is needed, including systematically evaluating outcomes and achievements.*

Wherever possible, nursing care plans should be jointly negotiated between the person with dementia, family members, nurses and other participants within the provision of care. Nurses need to help the person with dementia participate in care planning. The nurse needs to ensure that realistic and clear goals are outlined and that their responsibilities are clearly understood. The nurse needs to work alongside the person with dementia, their family and friends in systematically evaluating outcomes and achievements.

Making a Difference: *Facilitating access to and delivering the best quality, evidence-based, values-based health and social care interventions to meet the needs and aspirations of service users and their families and carers.*

Nurses working with people who have dementia should share with people who have dementia and their families and friends how to find out more about caring for people with dementia through the provision of services such as books, videos and the Internet, and through talk and discussion. The participation of people with dementia and families in support groups such as relative support groups should be encouraged.

Promoting Safety and Positive Risk: *Empowering the person to decide the level of risk they are prepared to take with their health and safety; this includes working with the tension between promoting safety and positive risk taking, including assessing and dealing with possible risks for service users, carers, family members, and the wider public.*

Nurses should enable people with dementia and their families to make decisions about the services they require. This will include helping them identify what activities and situations pose a risk to themselves and others and putting forward strategies that might reduce this risk. This will mean that nurses with work closely people with dementia and their family together with different agencies providing care. Nurses often need to help people with dementia, and sometimes their families, speak up for themselves and make choices about 'positive risk taking' (see Chapter 7).

Personal Development and Learning: *Keeping up to date with changes in practice and participating in life-long learning, personal and professional development for one's self and colleagues through supervision, appraisal and reflective practice.*

Nurses working with people who have dementia should keep up to date with changing views and approaches towards nursing people with dementia and their families. This may be accomplished by a variety of teaching strategies such as clinical supervision, ward-based seminars, workshops, conferences, educational and training programmes and through websites and discussion groups on the Internet. Through these means, nurses working with people who have dementia will come into contact with others who are providing care and will constitute a 'community of practice'. We believe that employing authorities should allocate part of their budget to training nurses to achieve good practice in relationship to people with dementia and their families.

We also think there is an increasing need for nurses to take responsibility for paying for their own education and training. This may not be welcome by many nurses who have been traditionally reliant on the NHS to pay for their training but as responsibility is gradually being transferred from the State to the individual within the United Kingdom, it is now appropriate for nurses to see Continuous Professional Development and its funding as primarily their responsibility. This is not such a bad thing though because nurses who take responsibility for their own training and educational needs will be able to ensure that it does happen and will be able to go on courses that they want to attend, which may be different from what their employers want them to do. Nurses should see paying for their own training and education as an investment, which will make them more marketable to employing agencies, will give them a better chance of choosing the jobs they want, and will offer them an increased opportunity of gaining promotion and attracting a better salary.

Competencies and Capabilities with Dementia Care Nursing

The idea of competencies and capabilities are combined in *'Best Practice Competencies and Capabilities for Pre-registration Mental Health Nurses in England'* (DH, 2006a). This document emerged out of the *'From Values to Action'* (DH, 2006) and draws on

- 'The Ten Essential Shared Capabilities for Mental Health Practice'
- The Standards of proficiency for pre-registration nursing education: First-level nurses – nursing standards of education to achieve the NMC standards of proficiency (Standard 7) (NMC)
- National Occupational Standards and National Workforce Competencies
- The Knowledge and Skills Framework (KSF)

We have amended the competences and capabilities outlined in *Best Practice Competencies and Capabilities for Pre-registration Mental Health Nurses in England* (DH, 2006a) and have set the skills required within dementia care nursing alongside the theory/evidence base which supports the use of the skill. These amended competencies and capabilities will allow nurses to link theory and evidence with skills required by dementia care nurses. These amendments are consistent with *Everybody's Business* (DH, 2005) and the whole systems approach developed in this book.

1. *Putting Values into Practice*
Competence
Promote a culture that values and respects the diversity of people with dementia and their families.

Theory	Skill
Theory to support the use of skills would include:

Theory relating to hearing the voice of people with dementia (Goldsmith, 1996), person-centred care (Kitwood, 1997), relationship-centred care (Nolan et al., 2004) and working within dementia care triads (Adams and Gardiner, 2005). | Work with people to create an inclusive culture that respects the dignity of people with dementia and their families through transparent decision-making.

Demonstrate an ability to work with a range of stakeholders to promote capacity for the inclusion of people with dementia. |

Also Chapters 8 and 9.	Encourage the active participation of people with dementia and their carer(s) to participate in care on the basis of informed choice.
	The ability to engage with families as equal partners in care.
	Present positive views of people with dementia and their informal provision of care by valuing their stories and life experiences.
	Demonstrate respect for people with dementia at all times, including the most vulnerable providing care that preserves personal dignity at all times.

2. *Improving Outcomes for Service Users*
Competence
Use a range of communication skills to establish, maintain and manage relationships between people who have dementia, their families and key people involved with their care.

Theory	Skill
Theory to support the use of skills would include: Theory about promoting good and effective communication and how it might be applied to dementia care settings (Killick and Allen, 2001). Also Chapters 8 and 9.	Be approachable, spend time with people who have dementia, understand and support their interests, needs and concerns. Demonstrate safe and effective use of interpersonal and basic counselling skills. Maximise brief, positive greetings or acknowledgement of others. Use of ordinary conversation with people who have dementia and their families that avoids professional jargon. Give feedback to others about clinical situations that is constructive and facilitates positive change.

3. Physical Care
Competence
Promote physical health and well-being for people with dementia and their families.

Theory	Skill
Theory to support the use of skills would include:	Identify and assess the physical needs of people with dementia.
Anatomy and physiology as it relates to older people including those with dementia.	Assess the capacity of people with dementia to maintain activities of living.
Maintenance of activities of daily living with people who have dementia (Hudson, 2003; Nay and Garrett, 2004).	Communicate with people who have dementia, groups and communities about promoting their health and well-being.
	Promote sexual well-being that is relevant and appropriate to the person with dementia and others.
	Undertake physiological measurements.

4. Psychosocial Care
Competency
Promote the optimum mental health and well-being of people with dementia and their family members and enable them to develop and maintain supportive social networks and relationships.

Theory	Skill
Theory to support the use of skills would include:	Promoting and supporting therapeutic engagement with people who have dementia within social networks.
Establishing therapeutic relationships.	Supporting people with dementia to use their rights and responsibilities.
The use and value of different activities and interventions with people who have dementia and their families.	Promoting useful and enjoyable activity.
The Mental Capacity Act 2005.	Access, plan, implement and evaluate evidence-based care.
Assessment and care planning in dementia care nursing.	Work in partnership with people who have dementia and their families.

Also see Chapters 7, 8, 9 and 14.

Appropriate use and response to evidence-based psychometric assessment tools.

Encouraging people with dementia and their family members to fully participate in the assessment, planning, implementation, monitoring and assessment of therapeutic interventions.

Facilitating joint decision-making between people with dementia and their family members.

Contribute towards achievable and meaningful goals from the view point of the person with dementia and family members.

Demonstrate the importance of advanced directives in setting mutual goals.

5. Risk and Risk Management

Competency

Work with people with dementia, their families and colleagues to maintain health, safety and well-being.

Theory	Skill
Theory to support the use of skills would include:	Demonstrate the application of appropriate legal and ethical frameworks to support practice.
Mental Capacity Act 2005.	
Risk	Support the health and safety of nurses, people with dementia, their families and society.
See also Chapters 7 and 14	
	Demonstrate the ability to work in partnership with people with dementia and their carers to promote privacy, dignity, health, safety and well-being.
	Work in partnership with people who have dementia to enable them to communicate their fears and knowledge of potential and actual danger, harm and

(Continued)

Theory	Skill
	abuse, particularly if their autonomy or learning ability is impaired.
	Promote, monitor and maintain health, safety and security in the clinical setting.
	Ensure all records are kept in line with local policy and procedures and stored according to the legal and regulatory requirements of data protection.
	Discuss implications and contraindications of all procedures with people who have dementia and their families.
	Obtain valid informed consent for all procedures, with attention to the special and exceptional needs of people with dementia.
	Recognition of signs and circumstances associated with aggression and violence.
	Demonstrate an awareness of prevention and risk-reduction strategies for aggression.
	Assess the level of risk and consider how the risks can be controlled to minimise harm.
	The ability to work as a member of the therapeutic team in making a safe and effective contribution to the de-escalation and management of anger and violence.
	Take immediate action to reduce risk when there is a danger to an individual's health, safety and well-being.

Assess people's risk of falls and implement evidence-based interventions.

Develop and agree individualised care plans with older people at risk of falls.

Maintain a safe, clean and welcoming environment.

Take immediate action where you find aspects of the environment are unsafe, unclean and unwelcoming.

Observe and monitor the general cleanliness of the environment and report to the appropriate person when there is concern over the level of cleanliness.

Identify hazards which could result in serious harm to people at work or other person.

Take relevant and timely corrective action to manage incidents or risks to health, safety and security.

6. A Positive, Modern Profession
Multi-disciplinary and multi-agency Working Competency

Work collaboratively with other disciplines and agencies to support people with dementia and their families to develop and maintain social networks and good relationships.

Theory	Skill
Theory to support the use of skills would include: Multidisciplinary and multi-agency work between people with dementia, family members and other professionals and agencies The development of specialist dementia care services. Social policy relating to older people and people with dementia.	Work effectively and assertively in a team, contributing to the decision-making process and taking responsibility for delegated action associated with the assessment, planning, implementation and evaluation of care. Clarify and confirm your role in the overall care programme and single-assessment process with people who have dementia and family carers.

(Continued)

Theory	Skill
See also Chapters 1 and 2.	Co-ordinate the integration of care for people with dementia working with team members and other agencies who impact directly, or indirectly, on the health and social care of the person with dementia.
	Ensure your contribution to the care programme approach and single-assessment process enables effective interventions to take place with an efficient use of resources.
	Modify your contribution to individualised programmes of care according to the agreements reached by the team.
	Encourage people with dementia to engage with agencies involved in their care, communicating the benefits for this and taking account of any legal restrictions

7. Personal and Professional Development
Competency

Demonstrate a commitment for continuing professional development and personal supervision activities, in order to enhance the knowledge, skills, values and attitudes needed to implement safe and effective nursing to people with dementia and their families.

Theory	Skill
Theory to support the use of skills. See Jasper (2006).	Using the clinical supervision and support systems available within and outside your organisation.
	Taking responsibility for your own personal and professional development, seeking and accessing developmental opportunities to enhance your provision of dementia care nursing.
	Use reflective practice, supervision and support to facilitate ongoing insights

into your emotional state and its impact on your work with people with dementia, their families and colleagues.

Set professional goals that are realistic and achievable.

Demonstrate key skills including literacy, numeracy and use of information technology.

Enable other workers to reflect on their own values, priorities, interests and effectiveness.

Delegate nursing care or associated tasks safely and appropriately.

Engage actively in peer supervision.

Summary

This chapter builds on the basic idea running through this book that nursing people with dementia and their families is something that nurses do and say. Initially the chapter examined the work undertaken in dementia care nursing in various clinical settings in which there are people with dementia. The chapter then moves on and examines different capabilities and competencies that nurses working with people who have dementia should possess and that promote the well-being of people with dementia and their families. The chapter argues that the competencies and capabilities that nurses use in dementia care settings cannot be understood without reference to theory and those skills are guided and directed by theory. While it is impossible to nurse people with dementia without skills, it is just as impossible to nurse people with dementia without an underlying theoretical framework that guides and directs the skills that are needed.

References

Abbey, J. (2003). Ageing, dementia and palliative care. In S. Aranada, and M. O'Connor (eds) *Palliative Care Nursing – A Guide to Practice* (2nd ed.). Melbourne: Ausmed pp. 313–326.

Adams, T. (1996). A descriptive study of the work of community psychiatric nurses with elderly demented people. *Journal of Advanced Nursing* 23, 1177–1184.

Adams, T. and Gardiner, P. (2005). Communication and interaction within dementia care triads: developing a theory for relationship-centred care. *Dementia: The International Journal of Social Research and Practice* 4, 2, 185–205.

Addington-Hall, J. (2000). *Positive Partnerships: Palliative Care for Adults with Severe Mental Health Problems.* National Council for Hospice and Specialist Palliative Care Services and Scottish Partnership Agency and Palliative and Cancer Care. Occasional Paper No. 17, London: Department of Palliative Care.

Albinsson, L. and Strang, P. (2003). Differences in supporting families of dementia patients and cancer patients: a palliative perspective. *Palliative Medicine* 17, 359–367.

Borbasi, S., Jones, J., Lockwood, C. and Emden, C. (2006). Health professionals' perspectives of providing care to people with dementia in the acute setting: Towards better practice. *Geriatric Nursing.* September/October 27, 5, pp. 300–308.

Butterworth, C. (1986). *Psychiatric Nursing in the Community, the Application of New Technologies to an Organisation in Transition.* PhD Dissertation, Birmingham: Aston University.

Capus, J. (2005). The Kingston Dementia Café: The benefits of establishing an Alzheimer's café for carers and people with dementia. *Dementia* 4, 4, 588–591.

Cantley, C. and Caswell, P. (2007). Assertive outreach and the CMHN: a role for the future. In J. Keady, C. Clarke and S. Page (eds) *Partnerships in Community Mental Health Nursing and Dementia Care: Practice Perspectives.* Buckingham: Open University Press. pp. 332–344.

Department of Health (2005). *Everybody's Business: Integrated Mental Health Services for Older Adults. A Service Development Guide.* London: Care Services Improvement Partnership (CSIP).

Department of Health (2006). *From Values to Action: The Chief Nursing Officer's Review of Mental Health Nursing.* London: Department of Health.

Department of Health (2006a). *Best Practice Competencies and Capabilities for Pre-registration Mental Health Nurses in England.* London: Department of Health.

de Vries, K. (2003). Palliative care for people with dementia. In T. Adams and J. Manthorpe (eds) *Dementia Care.* London: Arnold. pp. 114–131.

Fraser, S. and Greenwood, T. (2001). Coping with complexity: educating, for capability. *British Medical Journal* 323, 7316, 799–803.

Goldsmith, M. (1996). *Hearing the Voice of People with Dementia: Opportunities and Obstacles.* London: Jessica Kingsley Publishers.

Henderson, J. (2007). Palliative care in dementia: carers must be included. *Journal of Dementia Care* March/April 22–23.

Hudson, R. (2003). *Dementia Nursing: A Guide to Practice*. Oxford: Radcliffe Medical Press.

Iliffe, S. (2007). How others see us: general practitioner reflections on the role and value of the community mental health nurse in dementia care. In J. Keady, C. Clarke and S. Page (eds) *Partnerships in Community Mental Health Nursing and Dementia Care: Practice Perspectives*. Buckingham: Open University Press. pp. 25–39.

Jasper, M. (2006). *Professional Development, Reflection and Decision-making*. Oxford: Blackwell Publishing.

Killick, J. and Allen, K. (2001). *Communication and the Care of People with Dementia*. Buckingham: Open University Press.

Kitwood, T. (1997). *Dementia Reconsidered*. Buckingham: Open University Press.

Lindesay, J., Marudkar, M., van Diepen, E. and Wilcock, G. (2002). The second Leicester survey of memory clinics in the British Isles. *International Journal of Geriatric Psychiatry* 17, 41–47.

Lloyd-Williams, M. and Payne, S. (2002). Can multidisciplinary guidelines improve the palliation of symptoms in the terminal phase of dementia? *International Journal of Palliative Nursing* 8, 8, 370–375.

Mace, N. (2005). *Teaching Dementia Care: Skill and Understanding*. Baltimore: Johns Hopkins University Press.

Mackenzie, J. (2007). Ethnic Minority communities and the experience of dementia: a review and implications for practice. In J. Keady, C. Clarke and S. Page (eds) *Partnerships in Community Mental Health Nursing and Dementia Care: Practice Perspectives*. Buckingham: Open University Press. pp. 76–88.

National Audit Office (2007*). Improving Services and Support for People with Dementia*. London: National Audit Office.

National Institute for Mental Health in England (2004). *The Ten Essential Shared Capabilities: A Framework for the Whole of the Mental Health, Workforce*.www.scmh.org.uk/80256FBD004F6342/vWeb/pcPCHN6FRLDM

Nay, R. and Garrett, S. (2004). *Nursing Older People: Issues and Innovations*. (2nd ed.). Sydney: Churchill Livingstone.

NCPC/Alzheimer's Society (2006). *Exploring Palliative Care for People with Dementia*. London: NCPC.

NIMHE (2004). *The Ten Shared Capabilities: A framework for the Whole of the Mental Health Workforce*. London: NIMHE.

NMC (2004). *A NMC Code of Professional Conduct: Standards for Conduct, Performance and Ethics*. London: NMC

Nolan, L. (2006). Caring connections with older persons with dementia in an acute hospital setting – an hermeneutic interpretation of the staff nurse's experience. *International Journal of Older People Nursing* 1, 208–215.

Nolan, M. R., Davies, S., Brown J., Keady, J. and Nolan J. (2004). Beyond 'person-centred' care: a new vision for gerontological nursing. *Journal of Clinical Nursing* 13, s1, 45–53.

Norman, R. (2006). Observations of the experiences of people with dementia on general hospital wards. *Journal of Research in Nursing* 11, 453.

Page, S. (2003). From screening to intervention. In J. Keady, C. Clarke and T. Adams (eds) *Community Mental Health Nursing and Dementia Care: Practice Perspectives*. Buckingham: Open University Press. pp. 120–133.

Royal College of Psychiatrists (2005). *Who Cares Wins*. London: Royal College of Psychiatrists.

Scottish Executive (2006). *Rights, Relationships and Recovery*. Edinburgh: Scottish Executive.

Silverstein, N. M. and Maslow, K. (eds) (2006). *Improving Hospital Care for Persons with Dementia*. New York: Springer.

Williams, C. L., Hyer, K., Kelly, A., Leger-Krall, S. and Tappen, R. M. (2005). Developments of nurse competencies to improve dementia care. *Geriatric Nursing* 26, 2, 98–105.

Chapter 12

Social policy and relationship-centred dementia nursing

Liz Forbat

Learning Outcomes

By the end of this chapter you will be able to

- describe the differences between academic and practice issues in relation to social policy;
- identify the key policies related to caring and care relationships;
- relate these policies to the changing political contexts in which they were written;
- recognise the shortfalls of these policies in addressing relationship issues;
- describe the features of relationship-centred and systemically informed policy in relationship to dementia care nursing.

Introduction

Presently, practice models focus on the experience of the user. Increasingly, practitioners are identifying the need to move beyond the individual and to consider the complex web of relationships that support people in the community. Academic work and professional practice are increasingly drawing on systemic ideas such as those that have developed within family therapy, and can be considered systemically informed. This movement towards integrating ideas is, however, slow. Academia has had considerable time to develop theoretical and practical approaches to working with people in the context of their lives, relationships and support systems. Social policy, however, is still struggling to keep up with the changing theoretical models that have developed in academic settings. Policy is not geared up to respond to the wide range of identities and issues that occur in care relationships. This is the case in informal care, nursing and other forms of health and social care across different client groups, including people with dementia.

This is no surprise when one considers the very different businesses of academia, practice and policy construction. Within academia, many well-resourced and coherent models are produced by academics who are well versed in the field. These models are refined each year and are internally coherent but allow for complexity and contradictions with other theories. Within practice, a range of models are drawn upon to create a strong eclectic and integrative approach to nursing care. While some of these models may compete in terms of ideology or approach, in practice these issues are rarely of concern or even considered consciously by clinicians such as dementia care nurses.

For social policy, however, the aim is to develop a coherent body of frameworks that can inform practice. Contradictions across policy frameworks cannot be tolerated. Policy makers must strive to match the complexity of the academic base, with the diversity of actual practice, whilst achieving the policy goals that are guiding the government.

It is little wonder then that since person-centred care has entered nursing discourse, policy too has begun to weave such ideas into its current framework. Similarly, ideas of relationship-based policy that have arisen in academic contexts are beginning to be considered for inclusion within policy and practice (Henderson and Forbat, 2002; Nolan et al., 2003).

In this chapter, the policy backdrop of care is discussed with reference to informal (family) and formal care, connecting with issues of concern in dementia care nursing. The historical and political background to current policy and indicative trends are also described. The chapter ends with an overview of different ideas that could move policy, practice and theorising more in line with each other regarding the importance of understanding relationships and whole systems in dementia care nursing.

The United Kingdom Policy Context

Since Thatcher's leadership much social policy has been flavoured by neo-liberalism. The effect of this has been government's increasing withdrawal from interventionist approaches and a shift towards citizen autonomy and self-reliance.

In terms of care and people with dementia, the move away from interventionist government was visible in the priority given to informal care, with a particular growth in emphasis on community care. This was epitomised in a new framing of care services, within the *NHS and Community Care Act* (DH, 1990). This document outlined a new role for the State that underlined the importance of family carers and highlighted the need for the provision of professional domiciliary support within the community. This marked a move with service delivery from primary or secondary care settings into the community domain. One of the objectives of this policy was ostensibly to reduce costs incurred by the heavy provision of care services within institutional settings and to reduce the number of practitioners such as nurses required to undertake tasks that could be done by relatives or neighbours. It drew on ideas of responsibility and duty invoked by notions of family – calling on the rhetoric of traditional marriage vows 'in sickness and in health' and similar notions of interdependencies. This translated into discourses of family obligation to care for each other (Finch, 1989; Gilbert and Powell, 2005) and enabled large financial savings for the government as they no longer took responsibility for providing state care for people with physical impairments, mental health problems, intellectual disabilities and older people. This reignited previous academic debate about the differences between 'caring for' and 'caring about' (Bayley, 1973) that are proposed as different ways of conceptualising care, indicating both the instrumental and emotional components to caring relationships.

Since 1990 more legislation has sought to maintain and nurture the community provision of assistance within community/family domains. In England and Wales, the *Carer's (Recognition and Services) Act* (DH, 1995) was the first piece of legislation specifically and explicitly to address informal care, indicating the important status conferred on this group. It offers one core (though broad) definition of carers, which sets the scene for services to define and interact with people. The *Carer's (Recognition and Services) Act 1995* defines 'carers' as 'Adults (people aged 18 or over) who provide or intend to provide a substantial amount of care on a regular basis' (p. 2).

The objective of the 'Carer's (Recognition and Services) Act 1995' is to '[...] encourage an approach which considers support already available from family, friends or neighbours, the type of assistance needed by the person being assessed and how and whether the current arrangements for care can sustain the user in the community'. (DH, 1995a: pp. 1–3)

This second passage highlights the aim of the *Carer's (Recognition and Services) Act 1995*, which is to prioritise family (neighbours or friends) care over care provided by paid workers. The *Carer's (Recognition and Services) Act 1995* presents carers as lay members of the community who perform tasks for each other and, in doing so, require some degree of government-level recognition for the service they provide. The *Carer's (Recognition and Services) Act 1995* makes it possible for carers to ask for their own assessment – so they are awarded the same rights as the person receiving care, for example, in having their role and impact on life assessed and recognised. While there is not a statutory duty for services to provide additional help for the carer on the basis of the assessment, it indicates the government's stance of taking seriously the important, and at times demanding, role that carers perform in society.

The *Carer's (Recognition and Services) Act 1995* demarcates a conceptualisation of care that focuses entirely on instrumental tasks. These definitions of care, however, are quite stark in their failure to address the emotional or relational aspects of caring. Relationship issues are only hinted at in the practice guidance notes, and are framed as the potential for 'tension and conflict between users and carers' (DH, 1995b: p. 6).

Thus, while there is an indirect assertion that caregiving impacts on the carer, this is only in terms of ideas of stress or perhaps physical strain (back pain for example), rather than directly related to the relationship between carer and the person they care for.

Four years later, *The National Strategy for Carers* (DH, 1999a) constructed carers in a number of new and distinctive ways, offering 'carer' as a more complex and subtle role than in the *Carer's (Recognition and Services) Act 1995*. Close analysis of the opening three pages sees *The National Strategy for Carers* (DH, 1999a) treating carers as family members, as aware of their own identity as a carer, as co-workers and as commodities. These distinctions resonate with the different models offered by Twigg and Atkin (1994) who identified their role as resources, co-workers, co-clients and the superseded carer.

The following passage of *The National Strategy for Carers* (DH, 1999a) presents carers as being clients in their own right and with their own care needs. It joins with the rhetoric of the *Carer's (Recognition and Services) Act 1995* where carers were given specific recognition:

> Carers play a vital role – looking after those who are sick, disabled, vulnerable or frail. The Government believes that care should be something which people do with pride. We value the work that carers do. So we are giving new support to carers. Carers care for those in need of care. We now need to care about carers. (DH, 1999a: p. 11)

The opening paragraphs of the Strategy, including the one above, serve to develop a sense of joint responsibility of carers and a feeling that caring touches all our lives. In this way it begins to see caring as part of a broader system of support and relationships. *The National Strategy for Carers* (DH, 1999a) is explicit in positioning carers as performing an *essential* role for their family member, whilst preventing inappropriate strain on society's resources. The document offers some commentary on relationships, with the majority of space given over to constructing informal care as a highly valued and positive activity.

A critique of *The National Strategy for Carers* (DH, 1999a) by Lloyd (2002) pinpoints dissatisfaction with the over-simplistic way 'care' has been conceptualised. She also notes that the Strategy takes a partial approach by restricting understandings solely to the perspective of the carer – a feature common in care policy. The Strategy can be seen to contribute to the perpetuation of the polarisation of carer and person receiving care and gives little room to the reciprocal and multi-dimensional aspects of interpersonal relationships. Her critique, therefore, calls forth the need to attend to both sides of a care relationship, and indeed pay heed of the relationship itself.

Many other policy documents in England and Wales have also reflected the growing recognition of the importance of carers. As one example, the *National Service Framework for Mental Health* focuses on carers in Standard Six (DH, 1999b). What becomes clear in this document, and many other ways of talking about care, is that there is an assumption that care is a product – the provision of tasks, support and so on. This means that the medium through which care is provided – the relationship – is concealed. While it is common-sense that the care tasks need to be performed, it is the way in which they are done and the mediating relationship which service users most frequently comment on. This is particularly the case when care receivers describe troubled aspects to care (Rogers, 2005). However, while service users and caregivers themselves prioritise the importance of the relationship (Forbat, 2003), it is rarely, if ever, the focus of policy.

Recent policy has adopted a rather different tack. This is illustrated in *The National Service Framework for Older People* (DH, 2001a), which takes person-centred planning as a central plank in its approach to services for this client group. Standard Two focuses entirely on this and states that the NHS and social services should

> 'Treat older people as individuals and enable them to make choices about their own care. This is achieved through the single assessment process, integrated commissioning arrangements and integrated provision of services, including community equipment and continence services' (DH, 2001a: p. 23).

This paragraph indicates a laudable approach to thinking about the need for clarity in joint working between different commissioners and providers. The vision of person-centred care is a reaction against critiques of previous models of delivery which tended to represent a 'one size fits all' approach. 'Person-centred' care indicates a move towards tailoring services towards individuals' own assessed needs and circumstances.

Thus, person-centred planning has become a dominant organising principle for practice and policy approaches to care. However, despite much rhetoric and policy uptake of the importance of person-centred care, there is little evidence that people with dementia receive this (Sheard, 2004) or indeed that there is an evidence base for person-centred care or person-centred planning (Kinsella, 2000; Mansell and Beadle-Brown, 2004).

Other critiques of person-centred care are more conceptual (Adams and Gardiner, 2005). For example, while the opening phrase of the *National Service Framework for Older People's* (DH, 2001) treats people as individuals, this approach holds with it the potential to also treat people as intrinsically divorced from all the other interpersonal relationships and systems around them. To some extent the idea of 'individual' is pitted against the idea of 'person in relation to others'. As Nolan et al. (2003) have pointed out, this 'fails to account for the sorts of negotiations, interdependencies and reciprocities that characterize the best dyadic and triadic relationships' (p. 273). The authors go on to illustrate a departure from this terrain, with reference to *'Valuing People'* (DH, 2001b). They argue this policy is unique in recognising the need for a broad and inclusive approach to lives, which while being founded upon principles of person-centred care also draws on an idea of the importance of people in relation to others. Indeed, the document takes a very broad approach to understanding people's lives and the importance of the wide number of contexts which impact on people with learning disabilities. The policy has sections describing action for areas such as housing, travel and employment. One chapter of the document is given over to formulating an approach to working with carers, which would seem to underpin the essence of Nolan et al.'s (2003) point of service planning within broader networks of interpersonal support.

However, person-centred planning remains a central concern of the document, and it is, therefore, open to the same criticisms noted above regarding the lack of emphasis on the person-in-relation.

Not all policy has been tied up with person-centred approaches, however, and some are beginning to introduce ideas of joint working, indicating the importance of understanding the whole system in which care occurs. This created opportunities to develop working practices based on relationships and communication. Indeed the need for different systems and relationships to be acknowledged and improved has formed the basis to new assessment protocols across health and social care. The launch of the Single Assessment Process (SAP) has particular ramifications for the new ways that health and social care professionals work together. The SAP was introduced (in England and Wales) in 2001 as a component of the *National Service Framework for Older People* (DH, 2001a) and has been invoked in policy since, for example, *Everybody's Business* (DH, 2005). It is part of a broader drive to improve older people's services by encouraging and facilitating joint working and centralise the experiences of service users. The aim is to have only one assessment, which covers health *and* social care needs, rather than the previous system of similar assessments by different professionals. The outcome is one single-shared electronic record of basic issues and information.

Despite all the best intentions of policy makers to involve carers, to focus on the individual and to share information across professionals, there remains a gap in the way that services are conceived, theorised and delivered. This gap relates to the issue identified throughout this chapter – the need to recognise and respond to the relationships that are implicated and impacted on when there is a need for care.

The Case for a Relationship-centred and Systemically Informed Approach to Care Policy

While much dementia care is carried out by nurses and nursing assistants (and their community equivalents) a great deal is undertaken by partners or adult children in the person's home. Symptoms associated with dementia are not like those of other chronic conditions such as cancer or coronary heart disease; though each of these may necessitate facilitating medical interventions, personal care and life-style changes, they do not make demands on the carer to witness often vast personality changes, which may result in violent or verbally abusive acts. Dementia may involve not only the physical tasks of caring for someone but also seeing their personality and their essence seemingly change before their eyes, and with it, their understanding of their own relationship and how they relate to each other. For relatives and friends this has an immediate and important impact on how they see the condition. Indeed, changes in personality and loss of recent episodic memory fed into a dominant discourse of 'loss of personhood' within the academic literature and lay understandings. Such ideas are widely disputed now, and we know that the person and their identity is not lost, but is still very visible and obvious (Kitwood, 1997; Sabat, 2002).

For dementia care nurses who have not known the person for very long and rarely get to know of the person's biography, this notion of change in personality and presentation is largely lost. The impact of dementia on the relationship between the person with dementia and the nurse is muffled; they have had no prior relationship by which their current interactions can be marked against. This may explain why a 'relationship-centred' approach has had less emphasis than the more immediately meaningful 'person-centred' ideas. For the family carer, however, the relationship is often at the forefront of how, and indeed why, care is delivered. For family carers, then, there is a need not just to recognise that they play an integral part in providing assistance (as policy to date has), but to place relationships centrally within this understanding.

There is increasingly a need to understand care as something that occurs within a complex network of relationships and contexts, interlinking with a number of disparate organisations and institutions. It is no longer appropriate to consider dementia care nursing in isolation, ignoring relationships, family histories and services or future planning. This means that social and health care policy and practice reflects and works with the lived complexities of people's lives, resisting the temptation to distil such complexity into narrowly defined and understood categories of working and thinking.

What is needed is an informed understanding how different people and organisations interact. This is far from radical in its aims, but what is apparent in practice and academic settings is the limited extent to which this complexity is worked with.

It is an approach that is familiar within some practice traditions. Notably, family therapists have long since adopted and promoted a stance of working that is based on relational complexities and inter-connections between different people and processes within a system. This is known as systemic working. AFT-UK (the UK branch of the Association of Family Therapy) states that systemic work is based on the following understanding: 'The behaviour of individuals and families is influenced and maintained by the way other individuals and systems interact with them. This way of working involves engaging with the whole family system as a functioning unit' (AFT, UK, 2005).

Policy is just coming on board with these ideas. This is illustrated, for example, in the document *Everybody's Business* (DH, 2005) in what it calls a 'whole systems approach to commissioning integrated services' (p. 20). Though referring specifically to mental health and distress in older people, its approach has important implications for policy more widely. The document positions itself as reacting to an awareness of the complexity of care for older people and the need for an approach that includes the whole range of service providers. It describes an approach to commissioning that includes partnership working across all sectors, including statutory health and social care, the voluntary sector, independent sector and users and carers.

This document indicates that it can no longer be considered acceptable for care to be commissioned, performed and received in separate silos. There is a need for everyone to take up the mantle. This means no longer approaching dementia as a separately 'championed' enterprise. This new approach aims towards a position where understandings and treatment of mental illness in older people becomes 'everybody's business' and a true integration of best practice for all staff, and not just that of 'specialist practitioners'.

Everybody's Business (DH, 2005) is a positive step on the journey to partnership and joint working through its promotion of all staff being knowledgeable about all conditions. A whole systems approach is clearly a move in the right direction for services to be providing care that takes account of the myriad of influencing features and contexts. However, it is a long way from truly theorising, conceptualising or realising relationship-centred policy.

What Would a Relationship-centred and Systemically Informed Policy Look Like?

This section offers some ideas for re-shaping policy into a relationship-centred and systemically informed framework. The following offers an indication of what a relationship-centred approach to dementia might look like. This builds on systemic approaches, outlined and developed in Chapter 6. It draws on ideas from family therapy where the focus is directed towards how illnesses (and a whole host of other issues) impact not just the individual but also on whole relationship networks and systems. It is based on the idea that meaning is created out of context, and therefore to fully understand the impact of an illness such as dementia, one needs to consider the full range of contexts operating (Forbat and Service, 2005). This moves away from the individualist model proposed by person-centred care and towards an understanding of the interconnectedness of all aspects with a person's life.

An associated idea is to think of illnesses or conditions as located 'between' people rather than 'within' one person. This premise leads to a therapeutic approach that is less interested in pathologising individuals and more interested in learning how an illness impacts on relationships. It is this theoretical approach which could be usefully modelled and applied to policy.

Table 12.1 is an illustration which addresses the core question of whether dementia can be considered to be *located in a person* or whether it is *created between people*. It illustrates a systemic and relationship approach to understanding and working with people with dementia.

The left column offers a feature of dementia. Each subsequent column then offers a typical response on the basis of different approaches. The first grounds the example in the dominant biomedical model and outlines what the understanding and response would be from this perspective. This biomedical domain represents the epitome of understanding dementia as located within the individual as a result of individual neurology. The next column presents the current social policy response to the dementia symptom.

Table 12.1 Approaches towards dementia care

Dementia feature and response	Medical model understanding and response	Current policy response	Systemic/ relationship-centred understanding	
Wandering	Brain dysfunction resulting in challenging behaviour	Person-centred care in the National Service Framework for Older People; use of assistive technology (coordinated by the DH's Change Agent Team).	Understanding: The environment and system is troubled.	Solution: The person's relationship with their environment needs altering – make the environment calm, predictable, make sense, be structured, be suitably stimulating, and safe. Consider the context that relationships create.
	Solution: Sedative medication			
Memory loss	Neurological degeneration	Development and support of memory clinics for multi-professional screening. Informed by the Single Assessment Process.	Understanding: Relationships can help 'cover', 'mask' and 'save face' when memory fails.	Solution: Change the way people relate to each other, and encourage coping mechanisms between people.
	Solution: Medication, e.g. Aricept			

Table 12.1 (Continued)

Dementia feature and response	Medical model understanding and response	Current policy response	Systemic/relationship-centred understanding
Visual hallucinations	Brain dysfunction. Solution: medication to prevent/dampen hallucinations.	Importance of access to health care, e.g. National Service Framework for mental health.	Understanding: System can maintain and promote dignity. Solution: To understand the hallucinations as a form of communication. The hallucinations make sense within the person's framework and are interpretable through knowledge of current and past relationships.

Last, an illustration of what a relationship-based understanding and response might be is presented. This last column is not offered as a watertight re-theorisation of the whole of dementia care, but rather it is posited as a way of developing dialogue about the need not just for 'person-centred' care but also for 'relationship-centred' and systemic understandings of care.

It is worthwhile pausing for a moment to deconstruct some of these issues a little further to clarify how the relationship-centred approach differs from the current paradigms and models in dementia care. The case example of wandering is, within a biomedical approach, understood as being a difficult behaviour which is to be managed in some way. Often for busy ward staff, or pressured family carers, one response to wandering is to seek out medication that would somewhat sedate the person. While few people would argue this is the most appropriate response, often there is more emphasis on lack of staffing than there is on facilitating other approaches to wandering.

The current policy response is perhaps couched in the language of person-centred care. Here there may be an emphasis (guided by the Department of Health's Change Agent Team) on assistive technologies. For example, the use of alarms on external doors that would alert a carer if the person with dementia had left the building. The basic understanding of this, though, remains one of a problem to be solved, and largely positions wandering as a challenging behaviour.

A relationship-based approach to wandering, however, takes quite a different approach. Wandering is not pathologised, but is rather seen as an outcome of the relationship between the person with dementia and their environment. This takes the idea of problem away from the individual and places understanding of this behaviour within their environs. The aim of a relationship-centred approach is embedded in the need to understand how the person with dementia relates to their surroundings. The objective is to make things calm, predictable, make sense, be suitably stimulating and safe. Often what might be termed challenging behaviours are a result of failing to make the environmental context meet all these basic criteria. If the environment (e.g. garden or house) meets these requirements, the person will not move away from a safe area, and the need for alarms and other technologies may be significantly reduced (reference in Janicki and Dalton, 1999). Wandering can then be understood as meaningful to the person and a suitable and safe activity (Dewing, 2004).

The idea of relationship-based approach to practice and policy therefore is not necessarily about solely interpersonal relationships. It takes a very broad approach to understanding all the layers of context which influence and impact on dementia caregiving. It no longer associates illness as something that is located within one person; the symptoms are features to be managed by and within relationships.

Overall, a systemic and relationship-based social policy would have the following features (commensurate with systemic practice more generally). It would

- focus on the contexts and influences that impact on people's behaviours and beliefs;
- approach relationships from a very broad perspective;
- understand problems as mediated and experienced with relationships, rather than as located in people.

Summary

As noted at the beginning of this chapter, there is often a gulf between the academic models and theories that are developed, practice applications and social policy. While practice and policy seem to currently be focused on person-centred approaches, academia has been developing models which prioritise the relationship. This is based on an understanding that relationships are central to the delivery and receipt of all care, and that often the relationship itself is a form of care (Robb and Forbat, 2004).

Social policy needs to now move beyond an individualised understanding of what it means to be involved in a care relationship; it is time to grapple with the complexities of multi-layered relationships and contexts of care. This means relationships between all of the following people and systems: the person with dementia and their family, their paid-for carers/ professionals, the environment and social policy. It can no longer be thought adequate to view people with dementia in isolation. Years of social policy emphasising the needs and rights of carers has reinforced their important position on the nation's approach to care, but this falls short of connecting with the wider concern that relationships underpin not just care but everything we do. Without understanding relationships or the contexts in which we live, work and care, social policy and the nursing profession have barely scratched the surface of getting to grips with dementia.

References

Adams, T. and Gardiner, P. (2005) Communication and interaction within dementia care triads: developing a theory for relationship-centred care. *Dementia* 4(2): 185–205.

AFT-UK (2005) *http://www.aft.org.uk/* Accessed: December 1, 2005.

Bayley, M (1973) *Mental Handicap and Community Care*. London: RKP.

Department of Health (1990) *NHS and Community Care Act*. London: HMSO.

Department of Health (1995a) *Carer's (Recognition and Services) Act. Policy Guidance*. London: The Stationary Office.

Department of Health (1995b) *Carer's (Recognition and Services) Act. Practice Guidance*. London: The Stationary Office.

Department of Health (1999a) *Carers National Strategy for Carers*. London: The Stationary Office.

Department of Health (1999b) *National Service Framework for Mental Health*. London: The Stationary Office.

Department of Health (2001) *National Service Framework for Older People*. London: The Stationary Office.

Department of health (2001a) *National Service Framework for Older People*. London: The Stationary Office.

Department of Health (2001b) *Valuing People*. London: The Stationary Office.

Department of Health (2005) *Everybody's Business*. London: The Stationary Office.

Dewing, J. (2004) *Wandering and Older Persons with a Dementia: Developing a Method for Participation*. Paper presented at the Dementia Network Seminar Series, Edinburgh. April 28, 2004.

Finch, J. (1989) *Family Obligations and Social Change*. Cambridge: Polity Press.

Forbat, L. (2003) Relationship difficulties in dementia care: A discursive analysis of two women's accounts. *Dementia: The International Journal of Social Research and Practice*. 2(1): 67–84.

Forbat, L. and Service, J. P. (2005) Who cares? Contextual layers in end-of-life care for people with intellectual disability and dementia. *Dementia: The International Journal of Social Research and Practice*. 4(3): 413–431.

Gilbert, T. and Powell, J. (2005) Family, caring and ageing in the United Kingdom. *Scandinavian Journal of Caring Science*. 19: 53–57.

Henderson, J., and Forbat, L. (2002) Relationship based social policy: Personal and policy constructions of care. *Critical Social Policy*. 22(4): 665–683.

Janicki M. P. and Dalton A. J. (eds) (1999) *Dementia, aging and intellectual disabilities: A handbook*. London: Bruner/Mazel.

Kinsella, P. (2000) *What Are the Barriers in Relation to Person-centred Planning?* Wirral: Paradigm.

Kitwood, T. (1997) *Dementia Reconsidered: The Person Comes First*. Buckingham: Open University Press.

Lloyd, L. (2000) Caring about carers: only half the picture? *Critical Social Policy*. 20(1): 136–150.

Mansell, J. and Beadle-Brown, J. (2004) Person-centred planning or person-centred action? Policy and practice in intellectual disability services. *Journal of Applied Research in Intellectual Disabilities*. 17: 1–9.

Nolan, N., Grant, G., Keady, J. and Lundh, U. (2003) (eds). *Partnerships in Family Care: Understanding the Caregiving Career*. Buckingham: Open University Press.

Nolan, M., Grant, G., Keady, J. and Lundh, U. (2003) *New Directions for Partnerships: Relationship-centred Care*. In M. Nolan, G. Grant, J. Keady and U. Lundh (eds). *Partnerships in Family Care: Understanding the Caregiving Career*. Buckingham: Open University Press, pp. 257–290.

Robb, M., and Forbat, L. (2004) Introduction. In C. Malone, L. Forbat, M. Robb and J. Seden (eds). *Relating Experience: Stories from Health and Social Care*. London: Routledge, pp. 1–4.

Rogers, L. (2005) *This life: Community Care*. 8 December 2005. http://www.communitycare.co.uk/Articles/2005/12/08/52102/this-life.html?key=CARE

Sabat, S. (2002) Surviving manifestations of selfhood in Alzheimer's disease: a case study. *Dementia: The International Journal of Social Research and Practice*. 1: 25–36.

Sheard, D. (2004) Person-centred care: the emperor's new clothes? *Journal of Dementia Care*. 12(2): 22–25.

Twigg, J. and Atkin, K. (1994) *Carers Perceived. Policy and Practice in Informal Care*. Buckingham: Open University Press.

Chapter 13

Developing an ethical basis for relationship-centred and inclusive approaches towards dementia care nursing

Tula Brannelly

Learning Outcomes

After reading this chapter you will be able to

- critically discuss approaches towards ethics within dementia care nursing;
- explain how you might apply ethical approaches to working alongside people with dementia and their informal carers;
- identify how care can be negotiated and shared with others involved within dementia care nursing particularly, between people with dementia and informal carers;
- explain how you might use ethical approaches to reflect upon nursing practice.

Introduction

a concern with ethics is not about adding something to technical problems of knowledge and skill, but rather is about drawing out an inherent facet of practice. It is about making explicit that which is implicit ... . Thus members of the caring professions must be able both to give reasons for ethical choices and to be able to explain these in ethical terms. (Hugman, 2005: p. 29)

This chapter examines ethical issues for nurses working with people who have dementia and their family members acting as informal carers. Ethical care refers to good practice based on ethical values such as honesty, openness and trust. In dementia care many opportunities arise where nurses make decisions about care based on their values. Ethical considerations in nursing are often complex, involve many different people and frequently reflect the 'messiness' of care. Sometimes people's needs are overlooked and various issues such as lack of resources and inter-professional conflict may redirect the focus of care away from the person with dementia and their informal carers. Overlooking or not meeting the needs of the person with dementia and their informal carer means that the ethic is missing from care.

The approach adopted in this chapter is underpinned by social constructionism that argues that nursing practice is constructed by each participant involved in the provision of care. One implication of this position is that its construction is dependent on the ethics and value base of practitioners. In particular, this chapter examines how good ethical care is practised in dementia care nursing with reference to the way that nurses

▶ decide a starting point for what care is with people with dementia and their family members;
▶ include people with dementia and their family members within all parts of the provision of care;
▶ make decisions that are acceptable to the person with dementia and their informal carers;
▶ negotiate nursing actions with people with dementia and their family members;
▶ evaluate whether good care has been achieved.

Underpinning this chapter is the idea that there is a gap between the basic prescriptive rules governing nursing practice and the complex decision-making mechanisms that are necessary to care well. Broad prescriptive rules determine what action is available to the nurse when empowering approaches are no longer adequate. This dichotomy means that nurses are required to empower people, but when this approach is no longer effective, nurses have a duty to enforce care. In dementia care this can result in nurses having long-term relationships with people with dementia and their carers, fulfilling care as the person who has dementia and their carer require it, but when care can no longer be managed, the person with dementia is removed from their home, often without their consent, and this is accompanied by feelings of inadequacy by their carers. This chapter will discuss a number of ethical approaches drawn from different academic and professional disciplines within the context of providing good care to people with dementia and their carers. Finally, ethical principles are used to analyse an imagined narrative to examine how structured reflection can be used to understand how ethical care was provided and how it included the needs of the person with dementia, carers and nurses.

The Context of Dementia Care

Ethically difficult situations in dementia care nursing are different for carers than they are for nurses. Table 13.1 below identifies different ways in which carers and nurses look at ethics within dementia care nursing.

As nurses accumulate practice experience, situations that were initially complex become routine, and nurses accrue knowledge as they gain experience. In contrast, people with dementia and their

Table 13.1 Ethically difficult situations in dementia care

Carers	Nurses
Autonomy – people with dementia making decisions about the future	Capacity – deciding when someone is able to make decisions about the future (see Gunn et al., 1999)
Consent to medication or research	Conflict or difference between what the person with dementia and their family members want from care
Advance directives and whether they would apply in the future	Potential or suspected abuse
Research participation when confused or after death	Not knowing the preferences of the person with dementia
End of life issues, including euthanasia and physician-assisted suicide	Balancing duty of care when the person with dementia refuses care
Truth-telling – about issues such as recent bereavements	Educating carers
	Conflict or difference with other professionals

Source: Hughes, et al., 2002: p. 35: Brannelly, 2004: pp. 160–170.

carers often lack experience to know what is applicable and effective, particularly in the early stages of dementia when they do not know what to expect or how they will cope. Nurses and other professionals sometimes overlook the impact that this learning has on the relationships between the carer and the person with dementia and with professionals too.

Informal carers provide essential care for people with dementia and require an assessment of their needs so that nurses can help them continue providing care. Research into the lived experience of carers has primarily focused on their experience of burden. More recently, researchers have examined the benefits carers also receive from giving care and have argued that caring is not necessarily constructed by carers in the same way as it is by professionals (Barnes, 2006). Carers are often committed to fulfilling the most fundamental request that a person with dementia is likely to make, and that is to allow them to remain at home and not move them on to residential care (see Nolan and Dellasega, 2000). This commitment is not usually shared by other participants within the provision of care such as nurses, who commonly view residential care as inevitable.

The context of care is also changing. Nurses' roles have changed to encourage increased inclusion for users and carers within service provision, and the distinction between expert and lay person is no longer acceptable (Tschudin, 2003: p. 63). This means that nurses must do everything they can to help users such as people with dementia have a voice within the provision of their care. Because of the difficulties people with dementia have in relationship to their impaired ability to speak, it is important for nurses to help and encourage the person with dementia participate in every aspect of their care, not least when important decisions are being made.

Nurses need to see service users as 'experts' about themselves and their care; however, the nature of dementia means that nurses need to develop creative and imaginative ways of hearing the voice of people with dementia and facilitating their involvement (Goldsmith, 1996). There are fundamental questions about how people with dementia are informed and included in the provision of care that are often related to the distress dementia might bring to the diagnosis-bearer and their informal carer(s). This may be seen in the continued debate within dementia care about whether it is 'right' to tell someone their diagnosis and what can be done (Rice and Warner, 1995; Taylor, 1996). In addition, this is further complicated when we consider that the views and opinions of informal carers may or may not be the same as either those of the person with dementia or nurses.

Professional guidance falls short of providing adequate ethical responses for nurses to use in their work as they are unable to capture the complexities and messiness of situations that arise in practice settings. Professional guidelines provide very basic and broad prescriptions for avoiding abuse and neglect – but do not state precisely the exact nature of a particular nursing action. Rights too are based on the assumption of what cannot be done to a person. Moreover, nurses continually need to make decisions about whether the present care is adequate, sustainable and what the potential future options for nursing care are. Throughout, ethical care is required within the relationships that are established between nurses, people with dementia and their carers.

The Contributions of Ethical Theory to Nursing Practice

In recent postmodern thinking, ethics are considered situated and practised through relationships. Postmodern ethics are concerned with revisiting ideas developed in past eras such as Aristotelian ethics from the classical era and universalism from the modern era, and to consider their application to the practice of caring professions today (Hugman, 2005). Of particular interest within postmodern ethics is the decline of grand theory, the recognition of plurality, the idea of virtue as the basis of ethics, the role of emotions, especially compassion, and the importance of 'relational' aspects to ethics (pp. 1–7).

I surmised earlier that universalist principles fail to provide sufficient guidance. Instead, nurses within the context of postmodern ethics

- must look for difference rather than similarity when working alongside people facing similar difficulties;
- take each instance of practice and relationships with people as unique; and
- reflect on their reactions to how care was practised.

The emphasis here is on situated practice that examines the 'right' thing to do in that situation. Hugman (2005: p. 157) reminds practitioners of contemporary 'unsettling ethics': 'Compassion, care, sustainability, virtue, "being-for-Other" are all values that may count as primary, alongside duty, responsibility, fairness, justice and so on, without any one precluding consideration of another.'

This amounts to nurses working to provide empowering care, but then having to revert to duty of care or best interests when previous care is no longer adequate. The issue is whether it is possible to use a different framework to enable care beyond the earlier stages of dementia when tougher decisions are required, such as placement in residential care. The question, of course, is how to achieve this. I argue that ethical practice is better thought through using the principles of an ethic of care.

An Ethic of Care

An ethic of care (Gilligan, 1982; Tronto, 1993) is primarily a political argument for the de-gendering and de-privatisation of care (Sevenhuijsen, 2003), but has set out ethical practice upon which good care can be established. An ethic of care unpacks the process of care giving and receiving, recognising care as a human need (see Nussbaum, 2004). 'Care' is defined by Tronto (1993) as 'a species activity that includes everything we do to maintain, continue and repair our "world" so that we can live in it as well as possible'. The process of care involves both thought and action (Tronto, 1993: p. 108), and consists of four areas of practice (Tronto, 1993: pp. 102–105). These are caring about, caring for, taking care of and care-receiving (see Table 13.2).

Within this apparently simplistic presentation of care are found complex concepts based on the notions of value, dignity and respect for others. This framework accommodates the mix of providers that are usually involved in the care of the person with dementia as it may be lay carers who care about, whilst caring, giving and taking care of is attended to by practitioners rather than carers. The care-receiver tells us the quality of care.

Participation is facilitated through collaborative care. The emotional place, prescribed norms, rules and habits of practitioners, people with dementia and their carers are located in their collaborative relationship. An ethic of care emphasises care as a practice, that care is evident or not in the way that it is practised (Tronto, 1993: p. 126). These relate to an explicit understanding of all humans as givers and receivers of care – we are all dependent at some point in our lives on others to care for us. Nursing ethicists such as Gadow

Developing an ethical basis 249

Table 13.2 The practice of an ethic of care

Practice	Relates to
Caring about	seeing and recognizing care needs; paying attention to the factors which determine survival; having knowledge of particular care situations; understanding needs and choosing various strategies of action; culturally and individually shaped.
Taking care of	taking responsibility for initiating caring activities; having detailed knowledge of particular situations; seeing what is necessary in a given situation and employing the means necessary into action; involves notions of agency and responsibility.
Care-giving	direct meeting of needs for care; carrying out the daily routines and developing a thorough knowledge of them; 'repairing and maintaining the world' (Fisher and Tronto, 1990).
Care-receiving	The recipient of care will respond to the care received; provides the only way to know that caring needs have actually been met; the reactions of those towards whom care is directed; attention to these reactions is important for the quality of the care process.

Source: Tronto, 1993: pp. 102–108; Sevenhuijsen, 1998: p. 83.

(1996), Hess (2003) and Tschudin (2003) have considered how ethics are practised within interpersonal relationships between nurses and patients. An ethic of care builds on this to consider all potential care givers, providing all involved with a voice to direct care. There are four principles of an ethic of care, which are attentiveness, responsibility, competence and responsiveness (Tronto, 1993: 127).

Attentiveness refers to the ability of practitioners to grasp the needs of the person(s) for whom they provide care, as that person perceives them, to 'suspend one's own goals, ambitions, plans of life, and concerns, in order to recognise and to be attentive to others' (Tronto, 1993: p. 127). This requires the nurses to relinquish their (or perhaps their organisation's) agenda in the short term and focus on the need for care as the person experiencing it sees it. This perspective not only supports the voice of the person receiving care as the starting point for care but also recognises that care is needed by all and not just the person receiving direct care. This means that the needs of all involved, including those of the practitioner, are considered to find the 'right' way of providing care.

Responsibility moves towards a personal motivation for involvement to enable care. Nurses accept responsibility when they choose to act on the needs identified in 'attentiveness'. It is suggested that nurses' work moves beyond the stated minimum standards required by, for example, professional bodies, to a personal, and perhaps emotional involvement that is necessary to care well (Tronto, 1993: pp. 131–132).

Competence is evident in paying regard to the outcome or end result of the caring process. Therefore, 'intending to provide care, even accepting responsibility for it, but then failing to provide **good** care, means that in the end the need for care is not met' (Tronto, 1993; p. 133 emphasis added). Competence to care is directly affected by resources or the lack of them. Tronto argues that good care requires care outcomes to be defined by the care receiver, which presents difficulties for practitioners when people with dementia are unable to voice preferences. Working closely with the person with dementia and their carer (where there is one) in a trusting relationship to negotiate care outcomes is beneficial, especially where practitioners are involved over a long period of time. On the other hand, professional competence is associated with knowing limitations and protecting clients from risk (Nursing and Midwifery Council, 2004).

Responsiveness is a two-way process and allows the carer to 'consider the other's position as that other experiences it' (Tronto, 1993: p. 136). Responsiveness enables the practitioner to understand the person's experience, providing the opportunity when necessary to change care to make it more suitable. Where people with dementia are unable to verbally express satisfaction or dissatisfaction with care, nurses need to read non-verbal communication to understand the position of the care-receiver. This may need to be developed in discussions with family and friends and a biographical understanding of the individual enables practitioners to help reconstruct biography and provide better care (see Brannelly, 2004).

Reflection Using an Imagined Narrative

The principles and virtues within an ethic of care are useful for nurses working alongside people with dementia and their informal carers. Listening to what people want and ensuring that it is provided the way people want it may at first seem quite straightforward. Dilemmas, however, often arise when the person with dementia, their carer or their nurse or other care professional want diametrically opposed outcomes from care. When this occurs nurses need to ensure that they negotiate the nature of the care that is required which meets the needs of all. To illustrate how an ethic of care can be used to inform practice, I have brought together a story made up of elements of different situations that occurred for a number of people with dementia and the responses that were provided by community psychiatric nurse and social work practitioners when recounting the way that they had practiced. This was from a study of the facilitation of participation in care for people with dementia (Brannelly, 2004). I have analysed it using an ethic of care.

In all of the following cases there were differences in what practitioners, people with dementia and their carers wanted from care, usually owing to progression of dementia, which led to increased dependency and meaning that the carer was no longer able to provide care. In order to illustrate this I have created a hypothetical person with dementia and carer, and we shall call the person with dementia Ethel and her carer Bob.

Ethel was in her late 70s, lived alone and was moderately forgetful. She was referred to mental health care services by her son Bob, who was concerned that she was no longer eating well enough or able to cook and shop for herself. Bob and his children had been providing care to Ethel for about seven years before they thought that things were serious enough to contact her GP. During this time Ethel had been physically unwell with cancer and had been referred to an Oncology Clinic for treatment. Her Community Psychiatric Nurse (CPN) had been attending the hospital with her and was helping Ethel 'fill in the gaps' afterwards. Ethel was able to remember some of the consultation but required reminding what was said and clarification about what this meant.

> We dropped in and out of various things didn't we, and I remember yeah. I think she was testing the water a bit, she could take a little bit and then backed off and then could take a bit more ... I followed her lead. I felt I was following her lead. (CPN)

As Ethel's dementia progressed, practitioners were keen to reassure Bob that she was safe during the day and arranged for her to attend day care. She was receiving meals-on-wheels at home and someone came and helped her to get up and dressed in the morning. Bob, who lived nearby, visited twice a day and made sure that she was safe in the evening. At a case review meeting in the day centre, Ethel said that she was having problems with her daughter who was abusing her, and that they had always had a difficult relationship.

> When she started at the day services, I arranged a review meeting, so that was it, my involvement is finished now. And at the review meeting she started crying, and at that time the family was not involved, it was only the day centre staff and Ethel. She started crying and then we asked what happened, and this starting coming up, and I think for that review that day was more than two hours. That's how things started, so because of these other issues I couldn't close the case. I had to go back, I discussed with my manager and I had to go back, and again had another discussion with her. (Social Worker)

Shortly afterwards, Ethel showed signs of depression and stopped eating. In addition, she became very suspicious of paid-for carers who visited her and stopped letting them in. Moreover, she was experiencing side effects of her cancer treatment, which made her feel very uncomfortable. Bob was having his own difficulties too and was finding it difficult to cope because his child had a long-term illness. At a case conference that Ethel did not attend, it was decided in her absence that she should be admitted to a local psychiatric ward to treat her depression and provide the family with a break. Discussions about placements started to happen between different professionals involved in her care.

> I suppose it is difficult for her as well in the environment that she is in, if it is something that is going to make her very agitated then it is going to be very difficult for her to get settled. Her future residence isn't going to be ideal really. I think she was quite happy being at home, and that was what she wanted really, that was what she liked … . (CPN)

From this ward, Ethel was soon moved to a residential home for a trial period to see if she would accept it. In the event, she did not settle and was eventually taken home by Bob.

> So she would have had all day Friday, all day Saturday and Friday night there. And in fact she never went to bed the whole night. She just wouldn't get into bed. She was very, very unsettled, she was constantly saying I need to go home, where is my son, he's coming to take me home, can you ring him, I want to go home. And she was in a terrible, terrible state when he eventually turned up on the Saturday. And that was when we abandoned that. (Social Worker)

As a result of this failed attempt to place Ethel into a residential care home, more measured approaches were taken that allowed Ethel to actively contribute to the decision about what residential home she should go to. In spite of previous assumptions that Ethel did not know what was going on, it was realised that she did understand that Bob was struggling to care for her as well as his ill child. As a result of discussion that included her contribution, Ethel agreed to be admitted to a particular residential home for four weeks over Christmas with a view to seeing what she thought of it and perhaps stay on a permanent basis.

Her cancer was controlled by medication. During her four-week stay in the home, her physical condition deteriorated suddenly and Ethel became more dependent. The GP therefore arranged for her to move to another residential home without adequate assessment. Meanwhile her grandson died.

> I said, look something has happened, why is she falling, why this thing, why suddenly is she doubly incontinent. There must be something, I need to know that. There is no point moving her from one residential home to another residential home with this problem. They will come back after two days and say we are not coping. She has got all these issues right, either you need to sort these issues, and to find out why these things are happening before I move her anywhere else. And I didn't get any help that day. ... I felt really distressed that day honestly. I mean you are supposed to work as multi-disciplinary work, cooperative, collaboration. No it doesn't work. That day it did not work. It was needed that day but it didn't happen. (Social Worker)

Ethel's nurse, social worker and Bob looked at alternative homes for her, and found a nursing home that could look after her considering her increased needs. 'He [son] looked at the current home, and said he liked it, thought it was very nice and wanted his mom to go there. So it all happened very smoothly really, largely entirely a bureaucratic, administrative process really from then onwards' (Social Worker).

The nurse recognised the lack of involvement that Ethel had in her final placement, one which she appeared to be distressed about, as she constantly asked to leave and go back home. 'It is a dramatic thing to do to someone, their whole life is not as they knew it is, it is just fallen away from them' (CPN).

Using an Ethic of Care to Analyse the Practice Narrative

My aim here is not to comment on whether the practice was 'right' but rather to give worthwhile insights about what happened and discuss it in ethical terms. There are elements of inclusion throughout this account, and although the care provided does not follow the principles of an ethic of care completely, there are parts of it that incorporate those ethics. The purpose of this is to lead to a set of questions that nurses may use to reflect on practice so that when ethical dilemmas occur in practice situations, they may use these questions to guide and direct their ethical practice, and thereby avoid overlooking the needs and voice of any of the people involved.

Elements of Attentiveness

Practitioners, including the nurse, were attentive to Ethel and Bob in the following ways:

- Ethel remained at home until her placement in a psychiatric hospital. She was later involved in finding a placement that she liked.
- One practitioner talked about how she allowed Ethel to set the agenda for discussing her cancer and 'filled in the gaps' when Ethel could not remember what had been said to her in the previous day's consultation.
- The care that Ethel and Bob required was negotiated, both sets of needs were identified and practitioners worked sensitively with each of them to enable care to happen. This is illustrated when Ethel accepted placement at the day centre and agreed to residential care to give Bob an opportunity to care for his child.
- When Ethel presented family difficulties at the day centre review, the practitioner did not dismiss what she said but rather continued her involvement with regard to Ethel's support.
- Practitioners recognised Bob's needs and so Ethel had been admitted into hospital and later a residential home.
- Practitioners also were attentive to the fact that Ethel disliked hospital and residential care.

In contrast, it could be said that practitioners were inattentive when Ethel was moved to the residential home in which she had no involvement in the decision, as well as when the residential home she preferred was unable to continue caring for her and she was moved out to another.

So, attentiveness refers to nurses grasping the needs of the person but that no one person involved becomes the total focus of care.

Elements of Responsibility

- Ethel wanted to stay at home and home care was arranged to make this possible.
- Practitioners were responsive when Ethel's reaction to initial residential placement meant that they took her out of there and back home.
- When Ethel experienced significant changes in her functioning, her practitioner displayed a responsibility towards her and wanted to know what was happening to her. Importantly, the practitioner took a personal responsibility for it.

There was a lack of responsibility when other professionals involved in Ethel's care were unresponsive, such as the move to another residential home without her agreement. There was also a lack of responsibility when Ethel's placement was finalised and described by the practitioner as 'largely bureaucratic', signalling the end of the practitioner's personal involvement.

Responsibility is the way that practitioners act on the needs identified in attentiveness and are those identified by people involved in care. Nurses also need to care and have a personal motivation which demonstrates their commitment to making sure that care is implemented as is wished by people with dementia and their informal carers.

Elements of Competence

- When Ethel was able to remain at home, practitioners ensured that adequate care was provided to support her there.
- When Ethel's needs changed significantly, her practitioner wanted to find out what had happened so that she knew how to provide care next.

In contrast, despite understanding that Ethel was unhappy about her final residential placement, practitioners did not act upon this information to ensure care that was competent.

Competence is paying regard to the outcomes of care; this links with responsiveness, the next ethic, as practitioners need to listen to the care-receiver in order to act competently.

Elements of Responsiveness

- Ethel was happy at home and this was supported.
- Ethel accepted the placement at the day centre.
- The placement at the initial residential home was abandoned because Ethel did not like it there.
- Practitioners understood that Ethel was unhappily placed in the final placement (but failed to act on that).

The problem here is whether these were acted upon or not, and at times they were not for Ethel, so practitioners lacked responsiveness.

Having unpacked practice into the elements of an ethic of care, it is useful to discuss how this can be used to reflect on practice as it happens.

Providing ethical care is the potential to enable empowerment rather than oppression through practice. This applies to all involved in the care relationship, and the practitioner, by discerning all the agendas brought to that relationship, is able to deconstruct and consider whose agenda(s) are being met by the care that is planned. This means that practitioners listen to all involved rather than hearing one voice over another. In situations where negotiation is needed, it is often the voice of the person with dementia that is lost in these interactions. People with dementia are easily pathologised as confused, demented or incompetent and so become the easiest voice to lose in care.

Hugman (2005) noted the re-emergence of compassion as an important caring emotion. Having compassion for a person with dementia may mean to consider that person facing a placement that they do not want, against their will and with no alternative and no support from those around them (see Robb, 1967). Ethical care will have noted the person's wishes, negotiated care with them and worked at a rate where the person with dementia has felt able to lead and respond to care. Knowledge of the person is necessary to achieve this. As nurses are often involved over long periods of time in the care of the person with dementia, they are best placed to gather this knowledge and be part of decision-making processes that empower and not oppress. Finding the right path in these circumstances is often tricky. As Ethel's story illustrates, when straightforward care was required this was easily met – she was at home with a carer and support services. When Ethel's needs and Bob's needs increased, deciding what care was right became much more difficult. To help practitioners discern ethical practice I have identified six questions that nurses may find useful to unpack dementia care when deciding care is complex, so that all participants within the provision of dementia care are able to allow their voices to be heard and make choices that they want to make.

1. Do I know what the long-term and short-term preferences of all involved are?
2. If I make this decision in this circumstance whose needs am I meeting?
3. Have I considered the needs of all involved when reaching this decision?
4. Do the available resources allow me to provide the care preferred?
5. Will the care I provide be what the care-receiver wants?
6. What are the care-receivers telling me about the care they receive? Do I need to act on this to make the care better?

Summary

This chapter has discussed postmodern nursing ethics in the care of people with dementia and their informal carers. We would argue that this is an important area of professional and academic consideration in view of recent innovations in dementia care nursing, such as the development of relationship-centred and inclusive approaches. In addition, the chapter supports recent policy directives in the United Kingdom such as *Everybody's Business* (DH, 2005) that advocates development of a systems approach towards the care of older people with mental health conditions. Within this context, the chapter has brought together the theories of care and ethics from caring and political philosophies and applied them to dementia care. Using an imagined narrative, practitioners voices have been brought together to emphasise the way decisions are made about care. Questions have been provided that invite practitioners to think about ethics in the care they provide, particularly in ethically difficult and complex care situations in order to promote empowering rather than oppressive care for people with dementia and their carers.

References

Barnes, M. (2006). *Caring and Social Justice*. Basingstoke: Palgrave.

Brannelly, P. M. (2004). *Citizenship and Care for People with Dementia*. PhD Thesis. Birmingham: University of Birmingham.

Fisher, B. and Tronto, J. (1990). Towards a Feminist Theory of caring. In E. K. Abel and M. K. Nelson (eds.) *Circles of Care: Work and Indentity in Women's Lives*. New York: New York Press.

Gadow, S. A. (1996). Ethical narratives in practice. *Nursing Science Quarterly*, 9 (1), 8–9.

Gilligan, C. (1982). *In a Different Voice: Psychological Theory and Women's Development*. London: Harvard University Press.

Goldsmith, M. (1996). *Hearing the Voice of People with Dementia: Opportunities and Obstacles*. London: Jessica Kingsley.

Gunn, M. J., Wong, J. G., Clare, I. C. H. and Holland, A. J. (1999). Decision-making capacity. *Medical Law Review*, 7, 269–306.

Hess, J. D. (2003). Gadow's relational narrative: an elaboration. *Nursing Philosophy*, 4, 137–148.

Hughes, J. C., Hope, T., Savulescu, J. and Ziebland, S. (2002). Carers, ethics and dementia: a survey of the review of the literature. *International Journal of Geriatric Psychiatry*, 17, 35–40.

Hugman, R. (2005). *New Approaches in Ethics for the Caring Professions*. Basingstoke: Palgrave.

Nolan, M. and Dellasega, C. (2000). 'I really feel I've let him down': supporting family carers during long-term care placement for elders. *Journal of Advanced Nursing*, 31(4), 759–767.

Nursing and Midwifery Council (2004). *The NMC code of professional conduct: standards for conduct, performance and ethics*. London: NMC.

Nussbaum, M. (2004) Care, dependency and social Justice: A challenge to convential ideas of the social contract. In P. Llyod-Sherlock (ed.) *Living Longer: Ageing, Development and social protection*. Basingstoke: ZedBooks.

Rice, K. and Warner, N. (1995). 'How much do psychiatrists tell their patients?', *Alzheimer's Disease Society Newsletter*, May. London: Alzheimer's Disease Society.

Robb, B. (1967). *Sans Everything*. London: Nelson.

Sevenhuijsen, S. (2003). *Citizenship and the Ethics of Care Feminist Considerations on Justice, Morality and Politics*. London: Routledge.

Taylor, R. J. (1996). *Being Given a Diagnosis of Dementia. The Experiences of People with Dementia and Those Who Care for Someone with Dementia*. PhD Thesis. Milton Keynes: Open University.

Tronto, J. C. (1993). *Moral Boundaries – A Political Argument for an Ethic of Care*. London: Routledge.

Tschudin, V. (ed.) (2003). Narrative ethics in *Approaches to Ethics Nursing Beyond Boundaries*. London: Butterworth Heinemann.

Chapter 14

Dementia care nursing: the legal framework

Sue Hodge

Learning Outcomes

After reading this chapter you will be able to

- explain the basic principle of autonomy;
- outline the criteria imposed by common law to assess capacity;
- understand the requirements of the *Mental Capacity Act 2005*;
- be aware of the impact of the European Convention on Human Rights;
- apply the law to solve problems in caring for people lacking mental capacity.

 Introduction

This chapter seeks to explain why it is important for dementia care nurses, but also informal carers, to have some understanding of the legal framework within which care is delivered. It is not intended as a definitive account of all law relating to the delivery of health or social care but is aimed to alert the nurse to those aspects of the law which are of particular relevance, namely

- consent,
- the consequences of acting without consent.

It should be noted that the law which is discussed is the law of England and Wales. A brief introduction to the Scottish *Adults with Incapacity (Scotland) Act 2000* will be given at the end of this chapter.

What is Law?

A simple answer to this difficult question is that law provides an enforceable code for life. There is no aspect of life which is not in some way governed by the law. It provides or goes some way to provide

- a means to enforce agreements;
- a way to obtain compensation for injuries caused by others;
- an environment which is free from pollution;
- safety in the workplace;
- enforceable personal rights such as the right to live;
- and so on and so on. …

Although ignorance of the law is no excuse for breaking the rules, in reality everyone has to depend on textbooks, journals and lectures to explain what it is necessary to understand in a particular context – in the case of this book, in the context of the delivery of care to those suffering from dementia. Relevant law is found in a number of sources including

- common law,
- legislation (also known as statutes or Acts of Parliament) and delegated legislation (also known as statutory instruments, regulations or by-laws).

Case law is a means by which the judges explain what the law means and how it works in a particular case. Throughout this chapter references are given to various cases which are the authority on which the explanation is based. The importance of any particular decision depends on the status of the court hearing the case. In this regard, decisions of the Judicial Committee of the House of Lords (HL) or of the Court of Appeal (CA) carry the most weight.

The Relationship between Law and Ethics

As we have seen in Chapter 13, ethical principles and theories provide a useful tool to guide decision-making in relation to the delivery of care. It must be understood, however, that ethics can never justify or permit any action which is in fact unlawful. In the United Kingdom, ethics can influence the interpretation of law but can never override it. Actions must always be legal, but this does not necessarily mean that the actions will also be ethical (Insert 14:1).

Insert 14:1 Example

As you are walking in a local park, you see a child face down in a boating lake. Unless you are the parent of the child or actually responsible for it in some way, for example, the child's nanny, the law permits you to walk on by leaving the child to drown.

Common Law Provisions
Consent

The ethical principle of autonomy is reinforced and protected by law. The explanation usually quoted with approval by the judges comes from an American case in which Justice Cardoza said:

> Every human being of adult years and sound mind has a right to determine what shall be done with his own body; and a surgeon who performs an operation without his patient's consent commits an assault, for which he is liable in damages. (*Schloendorff* v. *Society of New York Hospital* 211 NY 125 (1914).)

While the position is on the face of it clear, the reality is not that simple. Issues which frequently give rise to concern include

- the information required to enable a person to make a decision,
- the capacity of that person to use that information to make the decision.

Information Giving

Before we can make any kind of decision it is important to be aware of the basic facts which apply. A person seeking consent to the delivery of care, whether a nurse or an informal carer, must give sufficient information to enable the patient to understand

- what is being suggested;
- why it is being suggested;
- what is actually involved;
- any side effects;
- alternatives, if any, including the right to disagree and/or refuse.

The explanation must be given in language which can be understood and questions must be fully and truthfully answered (*Sidaway* v *Bethlem Royal Hospital Governors* [1985]) 1 *All ER*

Problems arise in relation to the amount of information which must be given. While the general rule is that the patient must be given the information which a competent professional would consider necessary in the particular circumstances, issues of negligence arise when the patient alleges that consent would not have been given had the implications of the treatment or the risks attendant thereon been properly understood. It is in the area of attendant risk that some guidance has been given by the courts.

In *Sidaway* v *Bethlem Royal Hospital Governors* [1985] 1 *All ER* Lord Bridge explained English law must recognise 'a duty of the doctor to warn his patient of risk inherent in the treatment [proposed.]. … The critical limitation is that the duty is confined to material risk. The test of materiality is whether in the circumstances of the particular case … [a] reasonable person in the patient's position would be likely to attach significance to the risk'. (*Sidaway* v *Bethlem Royal Hospital Governors* [1985]) 1 *All ER* (Insert 14:2)

Insert 14: 2 Example

Mrs Sidaway consented to a spinal operation to relieve persistent pain in her right arm and shoulder. She had been warned of a 1% chance of things going wrong but not of the catastrophic nature of the potential harm. She alleged negligence in that the surgeon failed to warn her of the nature of that harm. Her claim was dismissed.

In *Chester v. Afshar* [2004] UKHL 41 Lord Hope, in paras. 48–59 concluded:

The function of the law is to protect the patient's right to choose. If it is to fulfil that function it must ensure that the duty to inform is respected by the doctor. It will fail to do this if an appropriate remedy cannot be given if the duty is breached and the very risk that the patient should have been told about occurs and she suffers injury. (para. 56) (Insert 14:3)

Insert 14:3 Example

Miss Chester experienced back pain and reluctantly agreed to surgery to relieve the pain. She was not told of a 1–2% risk of nerve damage. She had fairly severe nerve damage and alleged negligence in that she had not been informed of the risk. Her claim succeeded.

Mental Capacity

It is a well-established principle of both professional practice and the law that all adults are presumed to have the capacity to exercise their own autonomy and reach their own decisions. A recent case in which this principle was considered was *Ms B v An NHS Hospital Trust [2002] EWHC 429 (Fam)* in which Ms B sought a declaration that invasive treatment given to her was an unlawful trespass. Dame Elizabeth Butler-Sloss, President of the Family Division, granting the declaration, emphasised that a competent adult has an absolute right to consent to or refuse medical treatment for any reason. Her guidance can be summarised as follows:

- Mental capacity to consent or refuse treatment is to be presumed;
- A person with capacity has the right to have a refusal respected by the doctors;
- Issues as to capacity need to be resolved as quickly as possible but in the meantime treatment may continue;
- The consequences of the person's decision are irrelevant in deciding capacity;
- If the doctors concerned do not feel able to carry out the decision, they must refer the person to others who will respect the person's wishes;
- If the issue still cannot be resolved, application should be made to the courts.

Ms B had severe physical disability so that it could be, and perhaps should have been, anticipated that her capacity was unaffected and her decisions about her treatment would have to be respected.

In cases of mental illness where the patient is subject to section under the *Mental Health Act 1983* the issues may be less clear cut. Even in such cases, the presumption is that the patient has capacity in respect of all matters other than the mental illness which has led to the section. This is illustrated by the judgment of Thorpe J. in Re C (Adult: refusal of medical treatment) [1994] 1 All ER 819 when he explained that a person suffering from schizophrenia and subject to section under the *Mental Health Act 1983* who 'understood and retained the relevant treatment information, ... [who] in his own way believe[d] it, and ... arrived at a clear choice' was entitled to have his treatment decision respected.

When it is clear that a patient lacks capacity to make an autonomous decision, any decision made by the carer must be in the best interests of the particular patient in the particular circumstances. Thus in *Re F (Mental patient: sterilisation) [1989] 2 All ER 545* the court stated that to sterilise a mentally incompetent woman would not amount to battery in civil law as she would be seriously adversely affected by a pregnancy but she would benefit from freedom to lead a full personal life including sexual intercourse if she so wished. In the same case, general guidance was given as to what would constitute a patient's best interests, Lord Brandon stating 'The ... treatment will be in ... the best interests [of incapable patients] if, but only if, it is carried out in order either to save their lives or to ensure improvement or prevent deterioration in their physical or mental health.'

The legal justification for interference notwithstanding the patient's lack of capacity is argued to be the doctrine of necessity as '[o]therwise they would be deprived of medical care which they need and to which they are entitled' (per Lord Brandon in *Re F* cited above). It should not be assumed, however, that the doctrine of necessity provides a blanket authority to do whatever the carer believes to be in the patient's best interest.

The very real difficulty which faces dementia care nurses and informal carers professional or otherwise, is how the decision about whether a person lacks capacity or not should be made. In this area, as can probably be anticipated from the vague legal principles which have been outlined, the law is of little practical help.

Assessment of Capacity – General Rules

There is no single set of criteria which can be used to assess whether or not a person lacks capacity to make a decision. A simple test is that of status evidenced by the provisions of the *Mental Health Act (1983)* in relation to compulsory detention and treatment of certain persons suffering from mental illness. While such a test is acceptable in relation to those with serious mental illness, such an approach would be difficult to justify in other circumstances. The English approach has been to recognise that an 'individual may be competent for some decisions and not others', which ensures 'that the individual retains as much freedom and control over their life as they are capable of exercising' (Bartlett and Sandman (2005, p. 584)).

Most tests include a requirement that the person be able to manifest a choice. Should the ability to manifest choice be the only requirement? Although this would seem to be a simple and effective test, it is criticised by Buchanon and Brock (1986) as disregarding 'defects or mistakes ... present in the reasoning process leading to the choice'. This view reinforces a commonly held view that capacity equates with ability to reason, raising the possibility that *irrational* choices may be disregarded when capacity is an issue although the choices would be respected if made by others.

Bartlett and Sandman (2005) suggest that while simple decisions can be tested by the ability to manifest the choice, 'the nature or seriousness of the decision may have a role to play in the standard of capacity applied to it' (p. 588). If this is so, then a more complex test is required which takes account of the individual's evolving characteristics and values. To hold otherwise would exclude all earlier views that the individual might have had as irrelevant. Simple choice would, however, provide 'one unambiguous solution to the problem' (p. 589).

An alternative approach relates to an objective test which ignores reasoning ability and asks, instead, whether a reasonable person in the particular circumstances would have reached the same decision.

Since the Law Commission first reported on the difficulties relating to decision-making and assessment of capacity and proposed changes (*Law Comm.231 February 1995*), there has been a long consultation period culminating in the reforms made by the *Mental Capacity Act 2005*. It is not yet clear whether the changes will in fact provide the clear, unambiguous and comprehensive means to resolve issues of capacity and best interests which is needed.

The *Mental Capacity Act 2005*

The long-awaited *Mental Capacity Act 2005* came into effect during 2007. As will be noted, the Act largely repeats in statutory form the provisions of the common law which have been developed over centuries to govern decision-making, and which are outlined in the earlier part of this chapter. This means that the common law continues to be very relevant and provides guidance as to how the provisions of the Act are to be interpreted.

The Act is accompanied by a very detailed Code of Practice. By *ss. 42 and 43* of the Act, the Code has statutory force. Nurses working with people who have dementia and paid carers have a duty to have regard to the Code when acting in relation to a person who lacks capacity. The usual rule applies – any departure from the Code must be justified. (*R (on the application of Munjaz)* v *Mersey Care NHS Trust and Others [2003]EWCA Civ l036)*. Failure to follow the Code will be admissible as evidence in civil or criminal proceedings against a professional or paid carer.

What Does the Act Say?

The principles are found in Part 1. The basic presumption is that every person aged 18 or more has capacity – it is for those alleging lack of capacity to establish this fact. (*s.1(2)*.) The Act makes it clear that a person is not to be treated as without capacity

- until steps to assist him to make a decision have failed (*s.1(3)*);
- merely because he makes an unwise decision (*s.1(4)*).

Any act done must be in the person's best interests (*s.1(5)*) and must be done with the minimum restriction of their rights and freedom of action (*s.1(6)*).

The Test for Capacity

By s.2 ' ... a person lacks capacity in relation to a matter if at the material time he is unable to make a decision for himself in relation to the matter because of an impairment of, or a disturbance in the functioning of, the mind or brain'.

The Code states that a two-stage test is required:

i. Is there an impairment of or disturbance in the functioning of the person's mind or brain? If so,
ii. has it made that person unable to make the particular decision?

This is further explained in *s.3(1)* which states that a person is unable to make a decision if they cannot

- understand relevant information;
- retain that information;
- use the information or weigh it as part of the decision-making process;
- communicate the decision.

If there is no impairment or disturbance causing the inability to decide, a person does not lack capacity. Bartlett (2003) suggests

> The requirement of an impairment ... does ignore the possibility of an individual whose purely physical impairment results in incapacity. An individual without brain damage who falls unconscious following an accident [or some other cause] could be [an] example where inclusion within the ambit of disorder to the 'mind or brain' might tax language to the breaking point.

Decisions would still need to be made but such people are likely to be outside the ambit of the Act (Barlett 2003, p. 27).

The Code, in paragraphs 4.57–4.59, addresses the situation where someone refuses assessment. If the person is compliant and assessment is in their best interests, assessment can be made despite the refusal. Where an outright refusal is given, they cannot be forced to undergo assessment – the only route forward presently available is via the use of compulsory powers under the *Mental Health Act 1983*. This raises difficulties as a refusal to be assessed is not of itself evidence of illness permitting the use of compulsory powers.

Assessment of Capacity – Some Particular Problems

The writer is not qualified as a health care professional and is aware that her understanding of dementia is limited. Dementia is not one particular state which comes into being and automatically causes lack of capacity to make decisions. We have already seen that patients detained by virtue of the *Mental Health Act 1983* retain capacity in all other aspects of health and social care. One of the problems people with dementia experience is that it is a progressive condition which in the earlier stages may well leave a person with fluctuating mental capacity. This raises very real issues for dementia care nurses and informal carers. If the matter is not urgent, there is no doubt that the decision-making must be deferred until the person regains capacity. Problems arise when a decision has been made at such a time, but when it comes to be implemented, capacity has been diminished. The Code of Practice emphasises throughout that capacity must be *assessed at the time that the decision has to be made*. It is not legally possible for a person's capacity to be assessed once for all; capacity must always be reviewed from time to time taking into account the nature of the decision to be made.

Decisions in the Person's Best Interests

Once lack of capacity has been established, any decision which is made must be the least restrictive of the person's rights and freedoms and in their best interests. (*s.1(5) and (6)*.) *s.4* requires the decision maker to consider the following:

i. whether the person may at some time recover capacity and if so when;
ii. whether they can be helped to participate in the decision-making;
iii. the decision maker must not be influenced by any desire to bring about the person's death;
iv. what the person's past and present wishes and feelings are;
v. whether the person has made a written statement as to their wishes;
vi. beliefs and values which would be likely to influence the person's decision;
vii. other factors they would consider relevant.

By *s.4(7)* the decision maker is entitled to take into account and to consult, *where it is practicable and appropriate to do so*

i. anyone named as someone to be consulted on matters of the particular kind;
ii. carers or others interested in the person's welfare;
iii. the donee of any Lasting Power of Attorney (LPA);
iv. any deputy appointed by the court.

While the steps set out in *s.4* are worded as duties, it is clear that the Act does not provide an exhaustive list of what must be done and when the various issues are relevant. Each decision must be made on a case-by-case basis from the point of view of the person lacking capacity and taking into account all relevant circumstances (*s.4(2)*).

The most helpful, and perhaps controversial power given to the decision maker is the right to consult others. Families and informal carers may well take this as imposing a right to be consulted and to make a decision on behalf of the person lacking capacity. There is a widespread assumption that this already exists, which causes real difficulties where the views of the family and those of the nurse differ. Although it is important to consult those who are close to the person, it should be noted that the power to consult is not a duty imposed on professionals. It is limited to those cases where it is both *practicable and appropriate* to do so. This does not give a general discretion to decision makes as to whom to consult. Before confidentiality is breached, the decision maker must think carefully about whom to consult and be able to explain why a consultation which was carried out was both *practicable and appropriate*, and why a consultation not carried out was believed to be impracticable or inappropriate.

Once the rules have been followed, a decision maker will be protected if they reasonably believe that what is decided or done is in the best interests of the person concerned (*s.4(8)*). If the court is asked for a decision, formal evidence on which the decision is to be made is needed, but in other cases, the decision maker merely has to demonstrate *reasonable grounds for believing* that what is being done is in the person's best interests. If, with hindsight, the decision was wrong, this does not of itself mean that the decision was unlawful. However, an action for negligence and/or trespass to the person may be possible if reasonable grounds for belief at the time of the decision cannot be shown.

What is Covered?

Although the Act specifies that the acts must be in connection *with the care and treatment* of a person lacking capacity, this is broadly interpreted. The protection of the Act can extend to

- acts in connection with personal care;
- acts in connection with health care and treatment.

Although there is some debate over the issue, changing a person's residence is likely to be covered provided the Act is complied with. Adequate safeguards are to be provided by amendment of the Act as required by the *Bournewood* decision.

The use of restraint is governed by *s.6* which permits such use only when the person taking the action

i. reasonably believes that the restraint is necessary to prevent harm to the person lacking capacity; and
ii. the act is a proportionate response, in degree and duration, to the risk of actual harm and the seriousness of that harm.

Lasting Powers of Attorney

One of the major concerns for many people appears to be a fear that they will lose control over decisions which may be required in the future and that actions may be taken which they would refuse if able to do so. One way which is intended to alleviate this anxiety is the provision for the creation of a Lasting Power of Attorney (LPA).

These will replace enduring powers of attorney (EPAs) although the Act makes transitional arrangements to permit existing EPAs to continue to be used for the purposes for which they were originally made.

The LPA can be used to give a donee (D) authority to make decisions about

- personal welfare or particular aspects of welfare; and,
- property and affairs or specified aspects of these, including power to make such decisions if the person loses capacity(*s. 9(1)*).

There is always a possibility that D will exploit the donor or fail to act in the donor's best interest. Where concerns are raised, these can be reported to the Office of the Public Guardian who has powers of investigation and intervention (*s. 56*).

Advance Decisions to Refuse Treatment

The concept of a 'living will' has been around for some time. It is seen as a means whereby a person can make decisions today, while having capacity, about health care issues which may arise at a later time when capacity is lacking. If effective, this allows a person to exercise autonomy even after capacity to make decisions is lost or impaired. In reality, it should be noted that existing case law tends to demonstrate that a living will is unlikely to be effective as the amount of information on which it must be based to make it effective is more detailed than that which would usually be required by the general rules of consent. It is certainly possible, some would say probable, that the new provisions governing Advanced Decisions to Refuse Treatment (ADTs) will similarly lack effectiveness. You will make up your own mind in due course!

By *s.24* a person over 18 with capacity can make formal provision dealing with health care decision-making on his behalf if capacity is lost at a later date. The ADT can be effective even though the treatment is described in layman's terms (*s.24(2)*). It can be withdrawn or altered at any time. Alteration or withdrawal need not be written unless it relates to life-sustaining treatment (*s.24(5) and s.25(6)*) carers will need to be alert to ensure that wishes informally expressed are properly noted in the records, as this may be the only evidence available.

Provided ADT has been created in the appropriate manner, it will have the same effect if the creator loses capacity as a contemporaneous decision. It should be noted, however, that the powers relating to compulsory detention and treatment found in the *Mental Health Act 1983* will override the ADT in appropriate circumstances (*s.28*).

It may well be that the new provisions will not in fact simplify matters and it is certainly possible that the purpose of giving a person power to control their own treatment after losing capacity will not be fulfilled. Although the ADT is effective even if expressed in layman's terms, it will not apply if,

 i. the proposed treatment is not the treatment specified in the ADT;
 ii. the circumstances are not the same as those set out in the ADT;
 iii. there are reasonable grounds to believe that matters have changed (e.g. medical science has advanced) in ways which the person could not have anticipated and which would have affected their wishes.

Health care professionals must be aware that an ADT may exist and, if there are reasonable grounds to believe that it does exist and time permits, they must take reasonable steps to find out what the ADT says. The professional is responsible for considering whether the ADT is valid and if it is applicable to the particular treatment in the particular circumstances. Where dispute arises as to the effect of ADT, the decision must be made by the senior clinician after appropriate consultation. If there continues to be doubt or disagreement, application can be made to the Court of Protection.

Protection under the European Convention on Human Rights

Although the United Kingdom is bound in international law by the principles of treaties to which it is a party, such provisions can only have effect as part of UK law once formally incorporated by Parliament. An example of this, relevant to this chapter, is the

European Convention on Human Rights and Fundamental Freedoms 1952 (ECHR) which was largely brought into effect in England and Wales in October 2000 by the *Human Rights Act 1998* (HRA). HRA requires the courts to apply the ECHR to all cases which come before them and to take into account all the case-law of the European Court of Human Rights (ECtHR). ECHR imposes a number of duties on the State designed to protect individuals from abuse by the State or public bodies such as Health Trusts and Local Authorities. Individuals have a right to compensation for breach of their human rights.

Under *Article 5* every one has the right to liberty but by *Art.5(1)(c)* a person can lawfully be detained if,

   i. the individual is of unsound mind;
  ii. the basis for the detention is lawful; and,
 iii. domestic legal requirements must be met.

By *Art.5(4)* it is essential that the detention of a person under *Art.5(1)(c)* is subject to periodic review to ensure the lawfulness of the initial detention or its continuation. ECtHR has held that where review is not a requirement of domestic law, the person must be able to bring an action, whereby the detention is reviewed (*Megyeri* v. *Germany (1993) 15 EHRR 584*). The reviewing body must have power to assess the person's mental state and to order release if the criteria for detention are found not to be fulfilled.

In relation to people detained pursuant to the provisions of the MHA 1983, *Art.5* is fulfilled by the provisions relating to the Mental Health Review Tribunal and the requirement for continuing review. People who are in hospital voluntarily have the right to refuse assessment or treatment and to leave hospital when they choose to do so.

It is in the case of those who lack capacity to make their own decisions and who are acquiescent in their detention and/or treatment that difficulty arises. *Art.5* is breached as English law has no effective means to ensure that such detention is lawful in the first place nor that continuance is lawful in the second. *HL* v. *The UK* (2005) 40 EHRR 32 (usually referred to as 'Bournewood') involved the detention of a person with severe learning disability in a psychiatric hospital. As he seemed compliant, no steps were taken for his formal detention. The UK courts concluded that his detention was lawful. However the ECtHR held that the lack of a formal process to review the lawfulness of detention of acquiescent patients unable by reason of learning disability, dementia or some other cause to consent or refuse meant that detention and treatment was unlawful.

The judgment meant that future mental health legislation would need to take account of the fact that compliance does not necessarily indicate consent. Although Bournewood concerned detention in a psychiatric hospital, it is accepted by analogy that it applies to other forms of detention, for example, in a residential care home or nursing home. The *Mental Capacity Act 2005* has been amended to create protection sufficient to comply with *Art.5* discussed in the following paragraph.

Mental Health Act 2007

To deal with the Bournewood problem, Part 2 of the Mental Health Act 2007 sets out new procedures. A person who is at least 18 years, suffering from mental disorder and lacking capacity to consent to residence in a hospital or care home, can be detained in a hospital or care home provided it has been independently assessed that this is in the person's best interests, necessary to prevent harm to that person and proportionate to the risk of harm.

The Mental Health Act 2007 is likely to come into effect during 2008 and will be accompanied by a detailed Code of Practice. At the time of writing (August 2007) useful comment can be obtained from the Department of Health web-page.

Other Protective Law

While the most important area of concern for carers may well be the rules governing decision-making on behalf of those suffering from dementia, the person's interest need more protection than the civil law alone can provide. Unfortunately, not all carers are truly concerned with the welfare of the person being cared for and thus sanctions are needed.

A person who intentionally subjects another to abuse which causes physical or psychological harm can be convicted of various criminal offences ranging from assault occasioning actual bodily harm to attempted murder and punished accordingly. The real problem with such a charge is that the victim may well be genuinely unable to give evidence. While this can sometimes be overcome by the existence of corroborative physical evidence, for example the presence of bruising, many cases are likely to go unpunished for lack of evidence on which a conviction can be based.

This issue has been addressed by the *Mental Capacity Act 2005* which has created a new offence. By *s.44* a person who cares for someone who lacks or is believed to lack capacity (or who is acting under an LPA or EPA) is guilty of an offence *if he ill-treats or wilfully neglects* the person lacking capacity. The offence is punishable on summary conviction by imprisonment for up to six months and/or a fine and on indictment with a maximum of five years imprisonment and/or a fine.

The *Domestic Violence etc Act 2004, s.5* creates a new offence of causing or allowing the death of a child or a vulnerable adult. A *vulnerable adult* is a person over 16 years whose ability to protect himself from violence, abuse or neglect is significantly impaired through physical or mental disability or illness, through old age or otherwise. The definition of vulnerability clearly includes those suffering from dementia. The defendant must have been a member of the same household as the victim or must have had frequent contact with them at a time when there was significant risk of serious harm being caused to the victim such as in the case of grievous bodily harm. The defendant will be liable if he caused the death or allowed it to happen. In the latter case the defendant will only be guilty if

(a) he was aware or ought to have been aware of the risk;
(b) he failed to take such steps as could reasonably have been expected to protect the victim;
(c) the act occurred in circumstances of the kind that he foresaw or should have foreseen.

A person will be regarded as a member of the household if he visits so frequently that it would be reasonable to regard him as such. Punishment can be imprisonment for a maximum of 14 years and/or an unlimited fine.

The *Domestic Violence etc Act 2004* also requires a domestic homicide review when a person aged over 16 years has died as a result of violence, neglect or abuse by

a. a person related to him or with whom he has been in an intimate personal relationship, or
b. a member of the same household.

It is as yet far too early to assess the extent to which any of these new provisions will be of real protection.

Summary

The chapter has tried to identify relevant law, though of necessity has included more detail of the new legislation than anything else. This has largely been dictated by the lack of literature at present concerning the *Mental Capacity Act 2005* and the more recent final *Code of Practice* which was published in February 2007. The picture is still not complete as although the *Mental Health* Act 2007 has been enacted, the extent of the amendments to law cannot be fully understood until the Code of Practice is available, sometime in the latter part of 2007.

A Note on the Law of Scotland

As an English solicitor my knowledge and understanding of Scottish law is limited. I hope that the following paragraphs will suffice to indicate the scope of Scottish law relating to incapacity and enable the reader to seek more detail from appropriate sources.

Issues surrounding decision-making relating to welfare, financial and property matters by those lacking capacity are addressed by the *Adults with Incapacity (Scotland) Act 2000*. The Act is a complex piece of legislation which allows other people to make decisions for those who lack capacity. The basic principles governing all decision-making are found in *Part 1*:

- Any decision as to lack of capacity must be justified,
- Decisions must benefit the person.

The Act requires assessment of the capacity of a person to make a decision to be made at the time of the decision.

The Scottish Executive has produced separate Codes of Practice governing financial matters and welfare matters. Health issues are dealt with by the *Code of Practice for persons authorised to carry out medical treatment or research under Part 5 of the Act*. Immediate treatment to save life or prevent serious deterioration can be given where necessary; otherwise a medical practitioner must provide a certificate of incapacity. Separate certificates are needed unless it *would be unreasonable and impractical* to provide these. The Code of Practice gives the example of persons with dementia in a nursing home who have multiple health needs as well as a requirement for fundamental procedures relating to nutrition, hydration, elimination and so on (*Code of Practice at para.2.18*). The certificate lasts for a specified period of time which cannot exceed one year.

People can attempt to safeguard their own futures by means of power of attorney. Under *Part 2* of the Act this can take two forms, namely,

- a continuing power of attorney relating to property or financial affairs (*s.15*);
- a welfare power of attorney relating to personal welfare including most health care issues (*s.16*).

A useful summary of the law and sources of further information can be found in *Adults with Incapacity (Scotland) Act 2000: General Information* available at www.scotland.gov.uk/Publications/2006/03/07090322/0

References

Bartlett, P. and Sandland, R. (2003). *Mental Health Policy and Practice* (2nd ed.). Oxford: Oxford University Press.

Bartlett, P. (2005). *Blackstone's Guide to The Mental Capacity Act 2005*. Oxford: Oxford University Press.

Buchanon, A. and Brock, D. (1986). *Deciding for Others, Millbank Quarterly* 64 (Suppl. 2): 32–33.

DH/Care Services (2006). *Protecting the Vulnerable: The 'Bournewood' Consultation*. June, DH: London.

Hervey, T. K. and McHale, J. V. (2004). *Health Law and the European Union*. Cambridge: Cambridge University Press.

Scottish Executive *Adults with Incapacity (Scotland) Act 2000 Code of Practice for persons authorised to carry out medical treatment or research under Part 5 of the Act* SE/2002/73

Chapter 15

Where we are now and how dementia care nursing should move forward

Trevor Adams

Learning Outcomes

After reading the chapter you will be able to

- provide a summary of the whole systems approach within dementia care nursing;
- describe how the whole systems approach may be applied to theory, education, research and policy within dementia care nursing.

Developing the Whole Systems Approach to Dementia Care Nursing

The main concern of this book has been nursing people with dementia and their families. This is an important issue as there are increasing numbers of older people with dementia in Western society, and there are significant concerns about not only whether there will be enough people willing and able to provide their care but also whether these people will have sufficient knowledge and skills. The approach adopted in this book challenges institutional approaches to people with dementia that confine them outside mainstream society, institutionalise them within hospitals and care homes and contribute to their depersonalisation. It is ironic that while we have moved away from incarcerating people with dementia in large mental hospitals, many people with dementia now live in small care homes that are similarly isolated from the rest of society and who spend most of their time in mind-dulling inactivity. Perhaps not so much has changed!

I regret to say that many people's confidence in the ability of nurses to deliver good care to people with dementia is at a low ebb. I hear troubling stories about people with dementia not being fed, not receiving drinks, getting bruises and many more things that should not occur. I wonder whether some people suffer more from the effects of bad nursing care than from dementia itself! There are many reasons given for this epidemic of bad care, not least that nursing has become too theoretical, has lost its interest in practical care, and that nursing suffers from a shortage of cash and a lack of resources. This book shares these concerns about the deteriorating quality of nursing care to people with dementia. However, the book takes a more constructive and radical approach than just blaming the universities, the nurses and the NHS, and takes the view that underlying these issues are two fundamental issues: What is dementia care nursing? What needs to be done to make it possible?

To address these questions, the book develops a broad and inclusive approach towards nursing people with dementia and puts forward strategies for practice and policy within dementia care nursing. Underpinning the book is the sure and certain belief that nurses, given appropriate leadership and financial, educational and staffing resources are able to make an important and distinctive contribution to the well-being of people with dementia and their families.

The book acknowledges the problematic nature of dementia care nursing, for example, its past excessive medicalisation of people with dementia and its focus on either the person with dementia *or* their family carer, that highlights one and marginalises the other. Moreover, the book recognises that nursing people with dementia has often been subject to subtle and sometimes not so subtle forms of ageism from within the nursing profession. Often this is due to the contact, some though not all dementia care nurses have with taboo body fluids, such as urine and faeces. Thus, through its close and intimate work with people who have dementia, dementia care nursing is often seen as a form of 'dirty work' and through which nurses often find themselves marginalised. The book deplores this marginalisation of people with dementia and shows how through verbal and non-verbal processes that occur within and between families and nurses and other health and social care professionals people with dementia often find themselves excluded and disadvantaged. This can often be the precursor of physically and emotionally abused.

People with dementia often have a 'double vulnerability' as they not only have cognitive and sensory impairments but may also experience an 'excess disability' due to what other people say and do to them, and because of how society structures them. We hope that this book will focus the attention of all nurses working with people who have dementia, not only mental health nurses but also nurses working on general units, such as orthopaedic wards and accident and emergency units. We hope the book will stimulate a new professional and academic interest and commitment towards nursing people with dementia and their families.

The book argues that people with dementia, and for that matter family members and nurses too, are 'bio-psycho-social' entities and that nursing people with dementia should take full account of their physical, psychological and social experience and needs. Institutional approaches towards people with dementia care are underpinned by a warehousing approach and characterised by what Davies (2003) calls 'a controlled community'. This approach is concerned with performing routine physical tasks that leave people with dementia inactive and without social contact for long periods of the day. The book argues that to fully take account of 'bio-psycho-social' nature of people with dementia, dementia care nurses should address the holistic and interrelated needs of the body, cognition, emotions and relationships. We see this approach within the work of Tom Kitwood (1997) through his elaboration of his dialectical understanding of the dementia process. This means that mental health nurses need to take a broader view than just the psychosocial needs of the person with dementia and general nurses need to take a broader view than just addressing their physical needs. All forms of dementia care nursing are based on a dialectical view of the dementia process and are thus holistic.

This dialectical and holistic view of nursing people with dementia is seen in the way it is developed as an interactive human activity that is characterised by what is said and done to people with dementia and their informal carers. The book sees dementia care nursing as being concerned with promoting the physical, psychological and social well-being of the person with dementia and their family; mutually sustaining relationships through which meaning is co-constructed, about the physical and social world, and also subjective experience of it; and is linked to problems of everyday living that arise from someone having dementia. This understanding of dementia care nursing draws on the work of Professor Phil Barker, a leading authority in Mental Health Nursing, and we hope that defining dementia care nursing in this way will help establish a bridge between mental health nurses who specialise in people with dementia and other mental health nurses, and will help bring to an end the long-standing marginalisation of nursing people with dementia within mental health nursing and will promote cross-fertilisation of ideas between two areas of the same speciality.

The book highlights various key ideas that underpin dementia care nursing. These ideas are well-being, as the aim of dementia care nursing; reflection as a means of gaining insights, the body as the source of the dementia and a medium through which nursing care is given; voice, as a way people with dementia and their family members make their views and choices known to others, story, as a means that different versions of events are co-constructed and shared between different people associated with the provision of dementia nursing care and evidence, comprising accounts that particular versions of events have happened and different interventions are effective.

Over the past 20 years, critique of the excessive medicalisation of people with dementia and their care has led to the development of two different psychosocial approaches (Adams and Bartlett, 2003). The first approach highlights the experience of the person with dementia and includes person-centred care (Kitwood, 1997), and the second highlights the experience of informal carers. This book argues that the existence of two different approaches towards dementia care is problematic and has given rise to a dichotomous approach that highlights one major participant within dementia care and forgets the other.

Rather than taking an approach that excludes the interests of a particular participant, the book adopts a whole systems approach that recognises the interrelationship between different physical and psychosocial systems within dementia care comprising different people and agencies. Within this approach, communication is seen to occur within and between different biological, psychological and social systems that give rise to the construction of meaning, knowledge and identity and positions people with the social order and gives rise to differential power relations. The book sets this approach within a dialectical understanding of the relationship between physical/neurological impairment and social/psychological phenomena that gives rise to the dementia process and its consequences for the person with dementia and their family.

The book makes a substantial leap forward in developing theory about dementia care nursing and brings together aspects of dementia care that, since the 1980s, have become polarised. First, drawing on Kitwood's dialectical understanding of dementia, the book highlights the bio-psycho-social nature of dementia, in terms previously articulated by the World Health Organisation (WHO, 2002). Second, the book brings together approaches that highlight the continuing relationship between the person with dementia *and* their family carer(s) within a broader whole systems approach towards dementia care as advocated in health policy within the United Kingdom (DH, 2005).

Moreover, the book also moves thinking forward about how different systems interact with each other within dementia care. In Nursing, particularly contemporary Mental Health Nursing, there has been a tendency to vilify the medical model and to focus on psychological and social aspects of mental health care. This is no longer appropriate as dementia care nurses can no longer adopt an ideologically polarised position due to recent developments in medical diagnosis, genetics and pharmacology. Drawing on Critical Realism, the book provides a way nurses can incorporate knowledge about physical and material aspects of dementia care settings within a psychological and social framework, that it is hoped, will help erode the dualism that exists within Nursing that has separated mental health nursing from acute general nursing and dementia care nursing from other mental health nurses. The book draws heavily on conversation analysis and discourse analysis to show how within dementia care settings, communication occurs between different systems and gives rise to people's understanding of the world, its organisation and their experience of it (Potter, 1996). Underlying the book is a critique of the channelling model of communication that is commonly used to understand interaction in nursing (Berry, 2007). This model highlights the exchange of information between the sender and the recipient but does not take account of how the message may be changed by its context and how it is interpreted by each party. The model of communication developed in this book draws on Wittgenstein's position that language does not merely describe objects and events but rather structures, constructs and orders them. This means that people's experience of having dementia, being a relative or working as a nurse arises from different subject positions that are made available by what people are doing and saying within dementia care settings. It is in this way that dementia care nursing is socially constructed.

While we would certainly agree that dementia care nursing is socially constructed, we would also want to affirm that people, including people with dementia develop a sense of who they are by what they themselves do and say. This view challenges the 'Kitwoodian' view that the 'personhood' of people with dementia arises because of what other people do and say to them and recognises that not only do people with dementia make sense of situations but also that they are able to participate in decision-making and activities that allow them to be seen by others and themselves in a positive way. This view draws on the work of Archer (2000) and with respect to people with dementia, Kontos (2005). This view argues that the identity of people with dementia is acquired by what they themselves do and say, that is their practice or activity. This book would, therefore, argue that the identity of the person with dementia and their members of their family not only arises through what is said and done to them *but also* by what they themselves say and do. The book, therefore, recognises the importance of activity within the provision of dementia care nursing and reviews different activities that may be employed by dementia care nurses with individuals or families that promote their identity and well-being.

During the development of this book, the idea of 'recovery' was considered as a possible idea within dementia care nursing (Scottish Executive, 2006). The impetus for its inclusion arose from recent governmental reviews of mental health nursing such as *From Values to Action* (DH, 2006). After much consideration together with discussion with others, it was decided that while many ideas within the Recovery Approach were appropriate to dementia care nursing, there were substantial difficulties with the use of the term 'recovery' with people who have dementia and their informal carers. Despite the claim made in *From Values to Action* that recovery is not the same as cure, recovery is an important part of the discourse of medicine and is, thus, part of the same discursive framework as 'cure' (DH, 2006). We, therefore, believe it is not appropriate to use the term 'recovery' in many areas of dementia care nursing, and that its use in recent governmental reviews of mental health nursing displays a naivety about nursing people with dementia that may appear to some people as ill-informed and heartless. We would want to distance dementia care nursing from the idea of recovery and call upon

Department of Health and other governmental agencies to think much more thoroughly and gain more evidence about the applicability of the Recovery Approach to mental health nursing to people with dementia.

As dementia care nursing is a tangible and practical activity, the book identifies various capabilities and competencies that are required of nurses working alongside people with dementia and their families. As a means of linking theory and practice, the book argues that practical competencies and capabilities should be underpinned by a coherent theoretical base such as person-centred care, relationship-centred care or with respect to the present book, and the whole systems approach. Consideration of capabilities and competences is timely as there is a need to go 'beyond the talk and do the walk' in dementia care nursing and highlight practical aspects of dementia care nursing, such as the promotion of dignity and the provision of privacy. While the past 20 years has provided the opportunity to define, refine and disseminate important ideas like personhood and voice within dementia care nursing, it is now appropriate to implement and evaluate the application of these ideas and identify the capabilities and competencies that dementia care nurses should possess.

Drawing on a systemic approach, the book argues that caring for a person with dementia not only leads to emotional stress among family members but also gives rise to psychological distress among nurses. The book applies the idea of 'emotional labour' to dementia care nursing. The issue here is not so much whether emotional labour occurs but rather why it occurs and how it should be addressed. Kitwood (1997) points out that working with people who have dementia may develop defensive patterns of interaction that form a barrier between themselves and the person with dementia. Such approaches lead to institutionalisation and impairs the well-being of the person with dementia. The book suggests that NHS Trusts and nursing homes have a responsibility not only to provide managerial supervision but also to offer regular clinical supervision that helps nurses reflect upon and address situational and emotional aspects of their work. The book describes how clinical supervision may be implemented within dementia care nursing.

Whole systems approaches towards dementia care nursing raise legal and ethical issues that often focus on the rights of different people involved in the provision of dementia, including the person with dementia, to make choices and decisions. The problems with person-centred and carer approaches is that they only highlight the ability and right of one person to make choices and decisions. But what happens when the carer wants something different from the person with dementia? What right do different family members have to make choices and decisions? The inclusion of other people, with similar rights, raises issues about whose choices and decisions should prevail. The book has presented the recent legal position in the United Kingdom about people's mental capacity, namely that a person with dementia should be seen as having the mental capacity to make decisions, unless there is evidence to show otherwise. This principle has important implications for dementia care nursing. In addition, the book adopts a relational approach towards ethical decision-making within dementia care nursing of the family or even those of statutory agents, such as nurses.

The adoption of a whole systems approach not only acknowledges the contribution of systems outside the family and the provision of health and social care and suggest that people with dementia, families and nurses might join together in collective action with organisations such as the Alzheimer's Society and professional organisations such as the Royal College of Nursing to gain better services for people with dementia or challenging the National Institute for Health and Clinical Excellence (NICE) guidelines restricting the prescription of drugs that are likely to slow down the rate of confusion. Campaigns like these clearly show their ability to challenge government policy that seriously impairs the opportunity people with dementia have to maintain well-being. We would support such collective action and would highlight the close connection between what happens in government and the Department of Health, and the lives of people with dementia and their families. We would ask that a much clearer and transparent dialogue occurs between the Department of Health and all dementia care nurses about the future development of dementia care nursing.

To conclude, we support various recommendations that promote the development of good practice within dementia care nursing.

Theory

▶ Integration of person-centred and relationship-centred approaches within a whole systems approach towards dementia care nursing;

- Clarification about how the personhood of people with dementia, their family members and nurses arises not only from what is said and done to them but also by what they do themselves;
- Greater articulation about how communication between people and agencies within different systems constructs people's experience of having dementia or giving formal or informal care.

Practice

- Development of competencies and capabilities for dementia care nursing that are supported by theory and are applicable to a range of practice settings containing people with dementia and their families;
- Development of practice that promotes patterns of verbal and non-verbal communication that enhance the respect and dignity of people with dementia and enables their voice and choice to be heard and addressed;
- Integration into dementia care nursing of activities that promote the well-being of people with dementia and their families.

Education

- Increased undergraduate and post-graduate training about dementia care within pre-registration and post-registration adult and mental health nurse programmes;
- Increased number of professorial posts with an identified and specific interest in dementia care nursing;
- Better training in dementia care for nurses registered in other countries who are undertaking Overseas Nursing Programmes.

Research

- Increased funding from governmental agencies such as the Department of Health to develop the effectiveness of dementia care nursing through practice development programmes;
- Research that explores and develops a whole systems approach within dementia care nursing;
- Studies that identify the relationship between communication, activity and the identity of people with dementia and how it may contribute to the quality of dementia care nursing.

Policy

- Better consultation between practitioners and nurse academics and governmental agencies such as the Department of Health, CSIP and NIMHE about the future development of the speciality;
- The commissioning of a governmental report on dementia care nursing;
- Additional money made available to pay reasonable salaries to nurses working with people who have dementia and their families.

References

Archer, M. (2000). *Being Human: The Problem of Agency.* Cambridge: Cambridge University Press.

Berry, D. (2007). *Health Communication: Theory and Practice.* Buckingham. Open University Press.

Davies, S. (2003). Creating community: the basis for caring partnerships in nursing homes. In M. Nolan, G. Grant, J. Keady and U. Lundh (eds) *Partnerships in Family Care.* Maidenhead: Open University Press. pp. 218–237.

Department of Health (2005). *Everybody's Business: Integrated Mental Health Services for Older Adults. A Service Development Guide.* London: Care Services Improvement Partnership (CSIP).

Department of Health (2006). *From Values to Action.* London: Department of Health.

Kitwood, T. (1997). *Dementia Reconsidered.* Buckingham: Open University Press.

Kontos, P. C. (2005). Embodied selfhood in Alzheimer's: re-thinking person-centred care. *Dementia: The International Journal of Social Research and Practice* 4, 4, 553–570.

Potter, J. (1996). *Representing Reality: Discourse Rhetoric and Social Constructionism.* London: Sage.

Scottish Executive (2006). *Rights, Relationships and Recovery.* Edinburgh: Scottish Executive.

World Health Organisation (2002). *Towards a Common Language for Functioning, Disability and Health.* London: World Health Organisation.

Index